MANUAL OF TUMESCENT LIPOSCULPTURE AND LASER COSMETIC SURGERY

including
The Weekend Alternative
to the Facelift™

MANUAL OF TUMESCENT LIPOSCULPTURE AND LASER COSMETIC SURGERY

including
The Weekend Alternative
to the Facelift™

William R. Cook, Jr., M.D.
Kim K. Cook, M.D.
Coronado Skin Medical Center, Inc.
Coronado, California

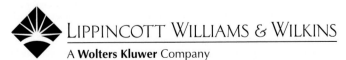

LIPPINCOTT WILLIAMS & WILKINS
A **Wolters Kluwer** Company
Philadelphia · Baltimore · New York · London
Buenos Aires · Hong Kong · Sydney · Tokyo

Acquisitions Editor: Beth Barry
Developmental Editor: Sonya L. Seigafuse
Manufacturing Manager: Tim Reynolds
Production Manager: Jodi Borgenicht
Production Editor: Deirdre Marino-Vasquez
Cover Designer: Mark Lerner
Indexer: Frances Lennie
Compositor: Maryland Composition

Cover: Henri Matisse, "Seated Pink Nude" 1935–6
© 1999 Succession H. Matisse, Paris/Artista Rights Society (ARS), New York
Slide courtesy Photo Archives Matisse

Printed and bound in China

9 8 7 6 5 4 3 2 1

Library of Congress Cataloging-in-Publication Data

Cook, William R., M.D.
    Manual of tumescent liposculpture and laser cosmetic surgery :
including The weekend alternative to the facelift / William R.
Cook, Jr., Kim K. Cook.
      p.   cm.
    Includes bibliographical references and index.
    ISBN 0-7817-1987-9 (hardcover)
    1. Liposculpture—Handbooks, manuals, etc. 2.
Liposuction—Handbooks, manuals, etc. 3. Surgery,
Plastic—Handbooks, manuals, etc. 4. Lasers in surgery—Handbooks,
manuals, etc. I. Cook, Kim K. II. Title.
    RD119.5.L55   C66   1999
    617.9´5—dc 21   98-50220
                                                        CIP

Care has been taken to confirm the accuracy of the information presented and to describe generally accepted practices. However, the authors and publisher are not responsible for errors or omissions or for any consequences from application of the information in this book and make no warranty, expressed or implied, with respect to the contents of the publication.

The authors and publisher have exerted every effort to ensure that drug selection and dosage set forth in this text are in accordance with current recommendations and practice at the time of publication. However, in view of ongoing research, changes in government regulations, and the constant flow of information relating to drug therapy and drug reactions, the reader is urged to check the package insert for each drug for any change in indications and dosage and for added warnings and precautions. This is particularly important when the recommended agent is a new or infrequently employed drug.

Some drugs and medical devices presented in this publication have Food and Drug Administration (FDA) clearance for limited use in restricted research settings. It is the responsibility of the health care provider to ascertain the FDA status of each drug or device planned for use in their clinical practice.

With great respect and love to our parents, Helen Cook and Roy and Kathy Krieger, for their invaluable support

CONTENTS

PREFACE

Humans have always dreamed of being able to perfect their faces and bodies in accordance with their own ideals. With tumescent liposculpture, we can come closer to that dream than ever before possible. Using a suction cannula to selectively remove fat deposits, surgeons can literally reshape the bodies of their patients.

In the early 1980s a procedure called liposuction was introduced to the United States from France. Since that time, liposuction has evolved and undergone significant changes. Dr. Jeffrey Klein introduced the most revolutionary change, a local anesthesia method known as the tumescent technique, which allows liposuction to be performed safely under local anesthesia with a quick recovery.

We have devoted our practices to refining and perfecting our individual specialties. Dr. William Cook has specialized exclusively in tumescent liposculpture and laser cosmetic surgery. Dr. Kim Cook has specialized in skin rejuvenation with an emphasis on laser peels. Together we have developed what is known as the Cook Weekend Alternative to the Facelift™, which utilizes a combination of our two specialties. This procedure redefines the traditional facelift by combining liposculpture, platysma muscle revision, and laser dermal resurfacing.

The *Manual of Tumescent Liposculpture and Laser Cosmetic Surgery* was written to provide information and instruction on the use of tumescent liposculpture under local anesthesia for practitioners of all levels of expertise. Also included are some of the latest procedures in laser cosmetic surgery. Of course, a description of a procedure cannot make a physician a great surgeon. Physicians must have a strong surgical background and specific hands-on instruction before attempting to perform this or any surgical procedure.

In this manual we describe the tumescent liposculpture technique, moving from one area of the body to the next, while focusing on the entire picture of what we call "Three Dimensional Tumescent Liposculpture™." We explain how the surgeon can go far beyond merely suctioning out excess fat in a two-dimensional approach. The surgeon who uses these techniques can become a true artist, shaping the patient's body in three dimensions. We also describe laser blepharoplasty, the Cook Total Body Peel, and laser skin resurfacing.

This book is not intended to be a verbose commentary with multiple case scenarios. Many people look upon manuals as "cookbooks" filled with "recipes," but there is no absolute recipe for a surgical procedure. However, techniques based on reproducible results can and do lead to successful surgical procedures and satisfied patients. The principles we outline in this manual have produced proven results in thousands of patients. Patient satisfaction is always the surgeon's goal. To achieve this the surgeon should aim to safely improve the patient's facial silhouette, body contour, and/or skin surface, while maintaining a natural, nonsurgical appearance.

ACKNOWLEDGMENTS

A text of this type is the accumulation of many years of experience and the influence of many colleagues. We are especially indebted to the late Dr. Garry Fenno, who as an early teacher and motivator of tumescent liposculpture laid the groundwork for Dr. William Cook's work in liposculpture. Fellow members of the Tumescent Liposuction Council, including Drs. William P. Coleman III, Rhoda S. Narins, Patrick J. Lillis, and Jeffrey A. Klein have been a continued inspiration over the years. We are grateful to our friend Dr. Gerald Bernstein for his review of this text and to Dr. C. William Hanke for his encouragement.

We sincerely appreciate the assistance of Roy Krieger, who helped with the proofing of the book; Melanie Nickel, for her countless hours and help in the composition and assembly of the text; and the staff of Coronado Skin Medical Center, Inc., for their support and help.

CHAPTER 1

ESTABLISHING A COSMETIC SURGERY PRACTICE

Training Requirements ▶ *Office Facility and Accreditation* ▶ *Staffing* ▶ *Tools and Equipment*

▷ Training Requirements

The surgeon performing cosmetic surgery should be a medical doctor who has received adequate training in dermatologic surgery, plastic surgery, otorhinolaryngology, or a related surgical field that provides preparation for technical surgery of this type.

Before attempting any tumescent liposculpture, the surgeon should take one or more approved courses that thoroughly present the procedure, the alternatives, and the risks. Hands-on instruction in performing the procedure itself is absolutely necessary. Regardless of how experienced one is in other surgical techniques, a definite learning curve is required to perform liposculpture with predictably good results.

Caution must be taken, particularly in the early stages of one's practice, to allow adequate time for the surgery and to follow the principles very carefully to achieve the best possible results.

It is helpful for the surgeon to be in good physical condition and have a good fitness and exercise program in place, so that he or she can meet the physical demands of this type of surgery.

▷ Office Facility and Accreditation

The facility where one performs cosmetic surgery procedures may be a clinical practice in which a portion of the office is designated as the surgical suite, a free-standing surgical center, or an accredited hospital. The staff should be knowledgeable about cosmetic procedures. A clinical office with surgical facilities provides a natural setting for cosmetic surgery. Ideally, the facility is comfortable and well-appointed, with a reasonably sized reception area (Fig. 1-1), consultation rooms (Fig. 1-2), a preoperative room, a surgical suite (Fig. 1-3), a postoperative recovery area, and a private exit from the facility.

When designing an office initially, it is helpful to follow the requirements of an accreditation agency, so that extensive renovations will not be necessary after the agency's inspection. Accreditation agencies include Medicare, the Accreditation Association for Ambulatory Health Care, Inc., and the American Association for Accreditation of Ambulatory Surgery Facilities, Inc. Relevant addresses are:

> Accreditation Association for Ambulatory Health Care
> 9933 Lawler Avenue
> Skokie, IL 60077
> www.aaahc.org

> American Association for Accreditation of Ambulatory Surgery
> Facilities, Inc.
> 1202 Allanson Road.
> Mundelein, IL 60060
> www.aaaasf.org

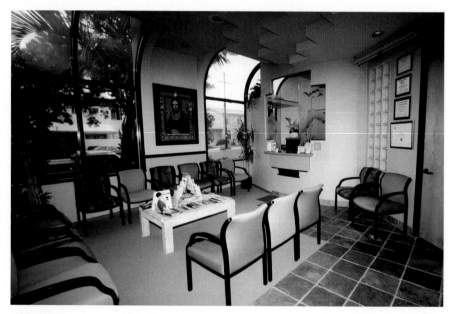

Figure 1-1
Reception area and waiting room.

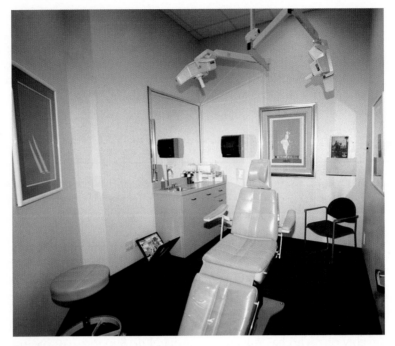

Figure 1-2
Consultation room.

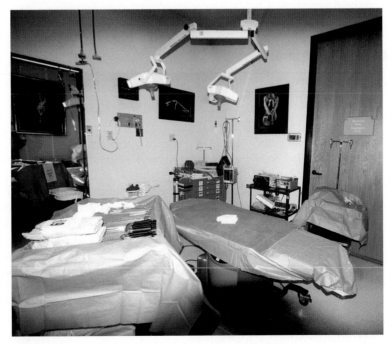

Figure 1-3
Surgical suite.

Accreditation is helpful for an outpatient surgery practice so that the facility is recognized not only as being approved, but also as providing a high quality of care. Accreditation gives the facility definite quality assurance protocols that are built into each and every surgical procedure, helping to assure consistently high standards. It should be noted that some states require accreditation as a prerequisite for any type of conscious sedation.

▷ Staffing

A surgeon's employees have an immense influence on the success of the practice. Every contact made within the office affects the patient's overall perception of the facility. Staff attitudes are especially important in a cosmetic surgery practice, where the patient's self-image is involved.

Cosmetic surgery produces many positive feelings for the patient, and a staff that appreciates this can make the experience even better. This applies to personnel at all levels: the receptionists, the nursing staff, and the business office personnel. Whenever possible, it is beneficial for the surgeon to personally review the candidates for each position to evaluate their skills.

The nursing staff should ideally include at least one registered nurse, preferably one who has Advanced Cardiac Life Support (ACLS) training and a surgical background sufficient to handle any emergency that might develop. Specialized training of the nurse(s) for one's own particular procedures will be performed by the surgeon and/or the existing staff. The facility may have a procedure manual, which is reviewed by each new employee.

▷ Tools and Equipment

The Operating Facility

The surgical suite should be of adequate size for the surgeon and several assistants to work comfortably (Fig. 1-4). A power table will be needed to position the patient according to the areas to be treated. Special comfort can be given to patients by use of the bodyCushion™ (Body Support Systems, see Appendix), a contoured cushion that makes it much more comfortable for those who have chronic low back problems. Adequate lighting and a good dedicated ventilation system contribute to an efficient operating facility. The surgical suite also includes instrument tables and adequate storage for medical supplies. A "crash cart" containing supplies and equipment for medical emergencies is vital to any operating room. Adjacent "clean" and "dirty" rooms are helpful for cleaning, washing, and sterilizing of instruments.

The Infiltration Device

Liposculpture using the tumescent technique requires an infiltration pump or other device to deliver the tumescent solution from the intravenous bag in which

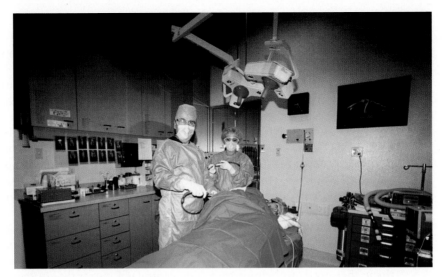

Figure 1-4
Tumescent liposculpture procedure underway.

it is traditionally mixed to the areas of the body undergoing treatment. After many years of experience, I have come to prefer the Klein infiltration pump, produced by the Wells Johnson Company. It provides a reliable method of delivering the solution to the appropriate areas at a controlled rate, which may be varied depending on the area being treated. Byron Medical and Bernsco Surgical Supply sell other similar infiltration pumps. See the Appendix for a partial directory of manufacturers of liposculpture apparatus.

The Vacuum Machine

Most surgeons use some type of mechanical device that produces a vacuum to aid in the removal of adipose tissue. Several companies, such as Bernsco, Wells Johnson, and Byron Medical, offer reliable, quiet machines that will perform for many years while requiring minimal service. For the surgeon who plans to do primarily liposculpture, a vacuum pump built into a separate room is recommended. This allows for a quiet and peaceful operating room, where the patient and staff can enjoy their favorite music.

I prefer using a mechanical vacuum machine, rather than aspirating by hand, because it allows me to concentrate on the process of sculpting the body. For myself, it is very distracting to have to worry about changing the aspirating syringe and other technical problems not relevant to the surgical procedure itself. The surgeon who uses an electrical vacuum pump usually has a backup machine readily available so that, in case the primary machine fails, the procedure can still be completed.

Cannulas

Small hollow stainless-steel tubes with variously shaped ends and a variable number of openings along the shaft are called cannulas.

These cannulas are used for the extraction of adipose tissue during liposculpture. Many types of cannulas are available to assist in body and facial contouring procedures. No one single tool will be suitable for every procedure and every surgeon. The surgeon has a variety of sizes and types of cannulas available from which to choose. This allows adaptation to varying conditions that may be encountered during a procedure, such as the thickness and density of the adipose layer, the amount of fibrosis, and the possible presence of cicatrix. To obtain the best results, the surgeon should be knowledgeable about a variety of cannulas and able to use them with precision.

In recent years, smaller cannulas have been developed that consistently produce excellent results. I recommend beginning a procedure with smaller diameter cannulas, and then increasing the cannula size according to the amount of fatty tissue that needs to be removed. The cannulas I currently use have diameters averaging 2 mm for the face and neck and 3 mm for body areas, with a range of 1.5 to 4 mm.

The Klein spatula-type cannulas (Klein Finesse cannula, Wells Johnson) have very small diameters (Fig. 1-5). I prefer to start and complete most body procedures using 12-, 14-, and 16-gauge Klein cannulas, in varying lengths depending on the area.

A variation on the Klein cannula is the Capistrano cannula (Fig. 1-6). This is similar in configuration to the Klein cannula, but has many small holes along a greater portion of the cannula. The Capistrano cannula works well in especially fibrous areas or areas of previous surgery.

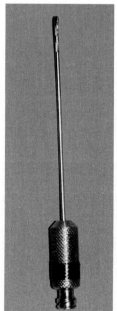
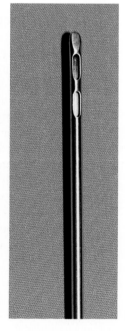

Figure 1-5

(**A**) Klein cannula. (**B**) Close-up of the tip of the Klein cannula.

A

B

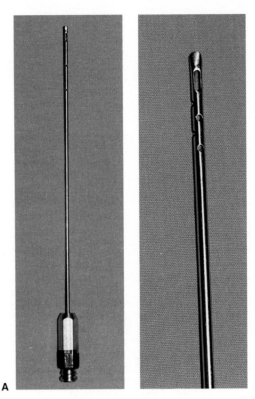

Figure 1-6

(**A**) Capistrano cannula. (**B**) Close-up
of the tip of the Capistrano cannula.　　　A

B

The Cook cannula (Fig. 1-7) is a very efficient open-ended cannula for almost any body area. This cannula is blunt, which makes it useful and safe for contouring curved surfaces. I also like the Cook cannula for sculpting the extremities, especially the arms and anterior thighs.

The Pinto cannula is open ended and rather pointed, which makes it penetrate fibrous areas more easily. For this reason it should be used only by more experienced surgeons.

I find the Klein and Capistrano cannulas best for sculpting the neck and face (Figs. 1-8 and 1-9). For most areas of the body, I prefer the Cook and Pinto cannulas (Fig. 1-10) for the majority of the suctioning, but also use the Klein and Capistrano cannulas. Both the Pinto and Cook cannulas are extremely efficient, producing a high yield and excellent results with less stress on the surgeon's arms.

In most body liposculpture procedures, I do the initial suctioning with a Klein spatula cannula, then switch to either a Pinto or a Cook cannula, gradually increasing the diameter up to 3 mm. The larger cannulas, such as 3.5 mm, are usually reserved for large-volume body reduction procedures. After completing the bulk of the suctioning, I finish the case by crisscrossing all areas with a fine Klein cannula, such as a 12 gauge. This helps to promote a smooth final surface.

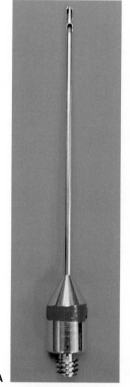
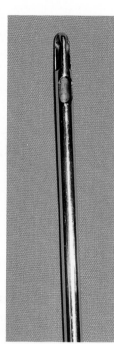

Figure 1-7
(**A**) Cook cannula. (**B**) Close-up of the
tip of the Cook cannula.   A   B

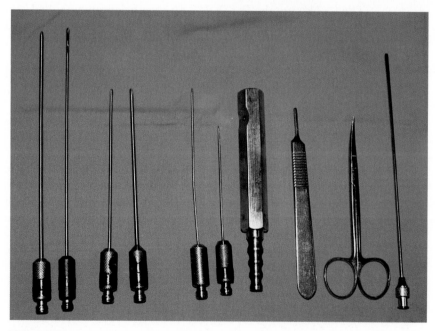

Figure 1-8
Typical surgical tray for liposculpture of the neck and face. From left to right, 6
Klein cannulas; cannula handle; blade handle; Iris scissors; and infiltration cannula.

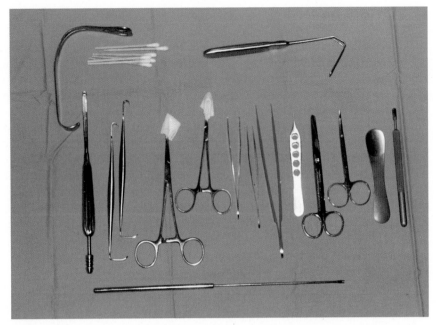

Figure 1-9

Typical surgical tray for the surgical component of the Cook Weekend Alternative to the Facelift™. Top, 2 retractors; from left to right, periosteal elevator, 2 retractors, 2 hemostats, 4 forceps, 2 scissors, Jaeger bone plate, pineapple metal surface; bottom, dissector.

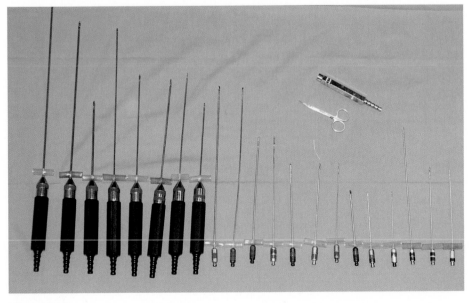

Figure 1-10

Typical surgical tray for body liposculpture. From left to right, 5 Cook cannulas, 3 Pinto cannulas, 10 Klein cannulas, 3 Capistrano cannulas; top, Iris scissors and cannula handle.

Waste Disposal

The liposculpture surgeon should be aware of the latest biomedical waste management regulations from both the federal and state Occupational Safety and Health Administrations (OSHA). Aspirated tissue is considered a medical waste, and therefore it must be disposed of properly through a licensed commercial waste remover such as BFI (see Appendix).

I collect the aspirated material in Baxter single-use plastic canisters. After they are filled, they are sealed in the office and then placed in red plastic trash bags, as mandated for biohazardous material. The bags are stored in a large 30-gallon receptacle, which is removed by the licensed waste remover. I prefer to collect the material in rigid canisters, rather than soft or bag-type containers, because the canisters are more reliable and more efficient for storing the tissue.

CHAPTER 2

ATTRACTING SUITABLE PATIENTS

Attracting Patients to the Practice ▶ *Patient Selection* ▶ *Points to Remember in Selecting Patients for Tumescent Liposculpture* ▶ *The Ideal Patient* ▶ *Patients to Avoid* ▶ *Contraindications*

▷ Attracting Patients to the Practice

Often, a surgeon who undertakes a liposculpture and cosmetic surgery practice is adding this specialty to an already existing practice. In that case, he or she has been performing other procedures that will have established a clientele in a particular area. When patients arrive at the office, they can easily be made aware that the surgeon is now performing cosmetic surgery. They can be educated about the procedure through brochures, books (Fig. 2-1), videotapes, or discussion with nursing staff. A small separate area or room in the office where the patient can view informational videotapes is very popular.

To gain additional patients from outside the office, we suggest presenting medical education seminars to provide useful general information. Use press releases to publicize the seminars in newspapers and regional magazines. Public relations in the print media are an excellent way to make patients aware of the surgeon, the surgeon's qualifications, and the procedures available.

By far the best method of attracting patients to a practice is referrals from other satisfied patients who have had surgery in the facility. If one attempts to be consistent and produces uniformly good results, one will have a steady flow of new patients who are suitable and pleasant to deal with.

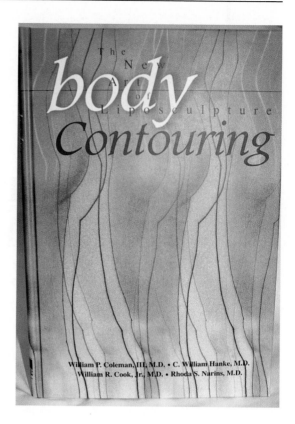

Figure 2-1
Book for patient education

▷ Patient Selection

With any cosmetic procedure, it is important to choose patients who are well suited for the procedure, both physically and psychologically. The interaction between patient and physician is very significant in any surgical procedure. The surgeon assesses whether the patient will benefit from the procedure and is seeking it for the right reasons. The patient should have confidence in the surgeon, realistic expectations, and an understanding of the benefits and potential risks of the procedure.

Patient selection has two aspects: the surgeon's criteria and the patient's expectations. The surgeon considers the criteria for choosing patients that he or she feels will gain the best results from the surgery. In order for the patient/surgeon interaction to be a success, thought is also given to the patient's expectations. Table 2-1 is a checklist of considerations that we consider useful in evaluating potential patients.

In theory, an ideal patient exists for any given procedure. However, in clinical practice one must consider many variables. Selection of appropriate patients is one of the most important aspects of a successful surgical practice.

TABLE 2-1 CHECKLIST FOR EVALUATING POTENTIAL PATIENTS

Surgeon		Patient	
Is the patient close to his or her ideal weight?	☐	What does the patient expect from the procedure?	☐
Is the patient physically fit?	☐	(Does the patient carry a photograph of a model or Hollywood star chosen to be his or her twin?)	
Does the patient have good skin and muscle tone?	☐	What is the patient's feeling toward cosmetic surgery in general?	☐
What is the patient's exercise program?	☐		
What are the patient's dietary habits?	☐	Has the patient had any unpleasant experiences with surgical procedures, either physical or emotional?	☐
Does the patient have any underlying medical problems?	☐		
Has the patient ever been diagnosed with any psychological or psychiatric conditions?	☐	Does the patient expect more than the surgeon can achieve with the surgical procedure?	☐
Has the patient lost excessive weight (over 100 lbs) recently?	☐	Does the patient want to become a different individual as a result of the surgery, or just to improve his or her physical appearance?	☐
Is the patient's body shape compatible with the final sculpting goal?	☐	Does the patient expect surgery to solve all the problems in his or her life?	☐

▷ Points to Remember in Selecting Patients for Tumescent Liposculpture

- ▶ Chronological age is not as important as apparent age.
- ▶ All ages can benefit, but limitations should be explained. We have performed liposculpture on patients from 15 to 85 years old.
- ▶ The patient's general health is evaluated.
- ▶ Skin tone and elasticity are evaluated, especially in the stomach, neck, arms, anterior thighs, and medial thighs.
- ▶ The patient's weight is compared to his or her ideal body weight. We have not performed liposculpture for morbidly obese individuals, and this book does not address unique surgical issues pertaining to these individuals.
- ▶ It is preferable that the patient's overall weight is stable. If the patient has lost 100 or more pounds in a short period, the skin will usually have lost much of its elastic contraction potential, so that the final contouring result may not be optimal.
- ▶ It is helpful if the patient performs at least moderate exercise. The patient who is motivated to exercise can generally achieve a more optimal result.
- ▶ Bone and muscle development are evaluated.

▷ The Ideal Patient

The hypothetical ideal candidate for liposculpture would be within 10 to 25 pounds of his or her ideal body weight and in good health. This ideal patient would have good skin elasticity, a balanced diet, and a regular exercise program.

Reasonable variations from this hypothetical ideal may be accepted. We have performed liposculpture on patients as young as 15 years old or as old as 85 years old, provided they meet the other criteria and understand the risks and limitations of the procedure.

Patients who are more than 20 pounds above their ideal body weight can benefit from liposculpture, especially if they maintain a stable weight and meet the other criteria.

Patients who are obese may benefit from the Cook Weekend Alternative to the Facelift™ (see Chapter 9) and from liposculpture of the arms (see Chapter 15). Their improved appearance following these procedures often motivates them to exercise and lose weight, therefore becoming better candidates for body liposculpture.

The ideal liposculpture patient seeks an improvement in his or her body shape, perhaps a more youthful contour, and better proportions. The ideal patient does not have unrealistic expectations that the procedure will dramatically change his or her life.

▷ Patients to Avoid

Patients who have recently lost large amounts of weight (100 pounds or more) are not ideal candidates for liposculpture because of poor skin elastic contraction potential and, usually, poor muscle tone. Recent weight loss of 50 to 100 pounds should be evaluated on an individual basis.

Patients who expect their bodies to be molded into a "twin" of some idealized person may be counseled, and perhaps avoided if they appear to have fixed, unrealistic expectations.

Patients who have a negative attitude towards cosmetic surgery or who were disappointed with previous cosmetic surgery results should be evaluated very carefully before proceeding.

Patients who are extremely unhappy with themselves and unrealistically expect the procedure to totally change their lives should be avoided. Their inevitable disappointment may cause difficulties for themselves and the surgeon.

Psychotic individuals must be evaluated carefully before accepting them as patients. A letter from the treating physician should be obtained. After surgery, they should continue with their psychiatric treatment and medications.

If a patient is in reasonably good health, but has an underlying medical problem, the primary physician can be consulted and his or her medical evaluation obtained before proceeding with liposculpture. For example, a patient who is on chronic corticosteroid treatment needs to be evaluated very carefully.

▷ Contraindications

Medical problems that may be relative contraindications for liposculpture include:

- ▶ Active untreated major cancer
- ▶ Major chemotherapy for active cancer
- ▶ Renal dialysis
- ▶ Active hepatitis or chronic liver failure
- ▶ Major immunosuppressive therapy
- ▶ Anticoagulant therapy
- ▶ Certain medications, possibly including some weight loss medications

The surgeon should always remember that this is an elective procedure. If there are questions that cannot be resolved, it may be better not to perform the surgery.

CHAPTER 3

INITIAL CONSULTATION FOR TUMESCENT LIPOSCULPTURE

Evaluating the Patient ▶ *Weight Factor* ▶ *Skin Tone* ▶ *Medical History* ▶ *Physical Examination and Body Analysis*

▷ Evaluating the Patient

The primary purpose of the initial consultation is to evaluate prospective patients and determine whether they are suitable candidates for liposculpture. At the same time, the initial consultation provides patients with an opportunity to learn what liposculpture can do for them and decide whether they wish to undergo the procedure.

Candidates should be evaluated with respect to their age (particularly their apparent age), weight, condition, general health, and skin elasticity (Fig. 3-1).

The surgeon should also evaluate the patient's reasons for seeking liposculpture and general psychological health. The checklist in Table 2-1 provides a good approach to evaluating the candidate for surgery.

▷ Weight Factor

Patients who maintain a stable weight for several months before surgery and who exercise regularly may be good candidates for liposculpture. However, one should be cautious about accepting patients who have lost a large amount of weight over

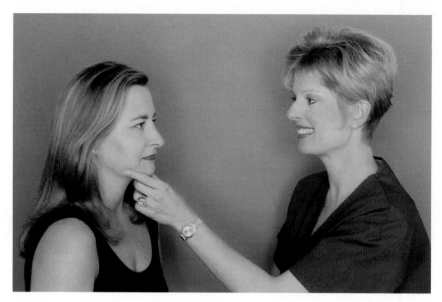

Figure 3-1

Dr. Kim Cook evaluates a prospective patient for the Cook Weekend Alternative to the Facelift™ and facial peel.

a short period of time; a weight loss of 100 pounds or more may lead to poor skin elasticity.

In general, I have not been performing liposculpture for morbidly obese patients, and this book does not address the unique surgical issues pertaining to these individuals. However, mega-liposuction is performed by some surgeons with good results. Please refer to other texts for more information on this procedure.

I generally recommend diet and exercise for obese patients. However, in some individuals who are considered to be too obese for three-dimensional body liposculpture, I may perform the Cook Weekend Alternative to the Facelift™ procedure (see Chapter 9) and/or liposculpture of the arms (see Chapter 15). This often improves an obese patient's appearance to such an extent that he or she achieves a more satisfactory self-image and gains the motivation to lose weight, thus possibly becoming a better candidate for additional liposculpture procedures.

▷ Skin Tone

Patients achieve the best results when they have at least a moderate amount of elasticity in their skin. Also, individuals who have good muscle tone from exercising appear to achieve better results from the procedure. Liposculpture will not remove striae distensae or scars. When carefully performed, it may produce some improvement in so-called "cellulite."

▷ Medical History

An evaluation of the surgical patient includes the patient's medical history, giving special attention to the following (for a more complete list of medical considerations, see Table 4-4):

- ▶ Bleeding tendencies
- ▶ Thrombophlebitis
- ▶ Previous surgeries
- ▶ Previous and current medications
- ▶ Infections
- ▶ Allergies
- ▶ Edema
- ▶ Emboli
- ▶ Psychiatric disorders

▷ Physical Examination and Body Analysis

If the patient appears to be a suitable candidate after initial discussion, a physical examination is performed. Body liposculpture patients should be evaluated in the standing position without clothes in the planned surgical areas. This allows the surgeon to see the effects of gravity while evaluating the patient's shape and planning his or her new contour.

The surgeon may perform a pinch test on the abdomen and other areas being evaluated (Figs. 3-2, 3-3). Patients must understand that it is not possible to suction fat that is intraabdominal. If a mixture of intraabdominal and subcutaneous fat is present, the patient should have realistic expectations regarding the degree of improvement that can be achieved from liposculpture.

During the physical examination, preexisting scars, hernias, asymmetry in muscle and bone development, overall weight, and skin tone are evaluated. Remember that one cannot give the patient a totally different body type. The bone and muscle structure of the body do not change as a result of liposculpture. In discussing possible procedures with patients, it is important to stress that the goal is body improvement, not perfection.

Specific points of physical examination and body analysis will be mentioned in each chapter. Two key areas to note on physical examination are the medial thighs and the knees. If the medial thighs have soft fat, patients must be warned that the skin might be loose after liposculpture. This area is extremely sensitive to removing too much fat. If one suctions the suprapatellar area of the knee without suctioning the entire anterior thigh, a step or line of demarcation will often result.

How many areas are to be suctioned? One very important consideration is the limit to the amount of lidocaine that can be infused in a specific patient (see Chapter 5). The surgeon's goal is to sculpt the appropriate number of contiguous areas so as to obtain the best three-dimensional figure possible for that particular individual. The surgeon should try not to suction too few or too many areas. The appropriate extent of liposculpture will be discussed in each of the corresponding chapters of the text.

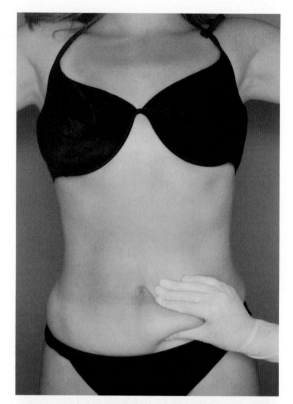

Figure 3-2

Prospective patient being evaluated for abdominal liposculpture. Note external subcutaneous fat layer.

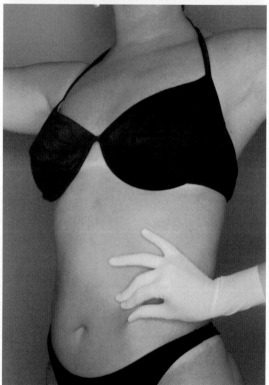

Figure 3-3

Different prospective patient being evaluated for abdominal liposculpture. Note absence of subcutaneous fat layer; abdominal protrusion is due to intraabdominal fat.

CHAPTER 4

PREOPERATIVE VISIT FOR TUMESCENT LIPOSCULPTURE

Goals of the Preoperative Visit ▶ *Physical Examination* ▶ *Laboratory Studies* ▶ *Medications* ▶ *Photography* ▶ *Surgical Garment* ▶ *Final Review*

▷ Goals of the Preoperative Visit

If the initial consultation is positive, we schedule a preoperative appointment with the patient. This preoperative visit provides a second chance for patients to ask questions, or to cancel surgery if they are unsure. During this visit, the procedure that is planned is reviewed and the alternatives, risks, and realistic goals are explained. Patients go through the surgical and other consent forms on a point-by-point basis so that they can obtain a complete understanding of the risks and expectations. Patients initial each point on the consent form. Our current forms include a surgical consent form for body liposculpture (Table 4-1) or facial surgery (Table 4-2) and permission forms for photography (Table 4-3), laboratory work, etc.

The medical history is reviewed (Table 4-4). Laboratory work is ordered and preoperative photographs are taken. Preoperative medications and an appropriate surgical garment are ordered. Required pre- and postoperative care is carefully explained. The patient is given written instructions regarding medications (Table 4-5), preoperative regimen (Table 4-6), and postoperative care (Tables 4-7, 4-8). In addition, the patient may be given a checklist of things to do before surgery (Table 4-9).

TABLE 4-1 PATIENT'S OPERATIVE CONSENT FOR BODY LIPOSCULPTURE

Patient name: _____

Patient states: I am aware that liposuction surgery (liposculpture) is a contouring process. Dr. Cook and assistants have explained to me the nature, goals, limitations, and possible complications of this procedure and alternative forms of treatment. I have had the opportunity to ask questions about the procedure, its limitations, and possible complications.
All items contained herein apply to the following procedure(s):
1. _____
2. _____
3. _____

I clearly understand and accept the following:
1. The potential benefits of the proposed procedure(s).
2. The possible alternate medical procedure(s).
3. The probability of success.
4. The reasonable anticipated consequences if the procedure(s) are not performed.
5. The possibility that additional services/fees may be required, including, but not limited to, anesthesia, laboratory, medications, and/or surgical facility or hospital use.
6. I will not drive for 24 hours after the procedure.
7. The goal of liposuction surgery, as in any cosmetic procedure, is improvement, not perfection.
8. There is no guarantee that the expected or anticipated results will be achieved.
9. The final result may not be apparent for 3–6 months postoperatively.
10. In rare instances to achieve the best possible result, additional procedures may be required. There may be a charge for any additional operation performed.
11. The surgical fee is paid for the operation itself and subsequent postoperative visits.
12. Strict adherence to postoperative instructions is necessary in order to achieve the best possible results.
13. Liposuction surgery is a contouring process and is not performed for the purpose of weight reduction.
14. Liposuction surgery does not guarantee the reduction of any measurements such as waist, neck, or any other area.
15. Areas of "cottage cheese" texture, so called "cellulite," will be changed little by the liposuction surgery.

Although complications following liposuction surgery are infrequent, I understand that the following may occur:
1. Bleeding is rare. In rare instances it could require hospitalization and blood transfusion. It is possible that blood clots or fluid may form requiring surgical drainage or medication.
2. Skin irregularities, lumpiness, hardness, and dimpling may occur postoperatively. Most of these problems will disappear with time and massage, but it is possible that they may persist permanently.
3. If loose skin is present in the treated areas, it may or may not shrink to conform to the new contour.
4. Infection is rare, but should it occur, treatment with antibiotics and/or surgical drainage may be required.
5. Possible numbness or increased sensitivity of the skin over treated areas may persist for months, and in rare cases may be permanent.
6. .Objectionable bruising, scarring, or pigmentation is rare, but it is possible.
7. Dizziness may occur following liposuction surgery, particularly upon rising from a lying or sitting position. If dizziness occurs, exercise caution while walking and do not attempt to drive a car.
8. Allergic or toxic responses to anesthesia are extremely rare, but possible.
9. In addition to these possible complications, I am aware of the general risks inherent in all surgical procedures and administration of anesthetic.

continued

TABLE 4-1 Continued

My signature certifies that I have discussed the above material thoroughly with Dr. Cook and assistants. I understand the goals, limitations, and possible complications of liposuction surgery. I wish to proceed with the operation. I authorize and direct Dr. Cook and/or associates or assistants of his choice to perform liposuction surgery on me and/or to do any other additional therapeutic procedure that his judgment may dictate to be advisable, reasonable, or necessary for my well being.

Patient signature: _____ Date _____
Witness signature: _____ Date _____
Physician signature: _____ Date _____

TABLE 4-2 PATIENT'S OPERATIVE CONSENT FOR FACIAL SURGERY (THE COOK WEEKEND ALTERNATIVE TO THE FACELIFT™)

Patient name: _____

Patient states: I am aware that the Cook Weekend Alternative to the Facelift™ (including but not limited to liposculpture, platysma muscle revision, laser dermal resurfacing, etc.) is a contouring process. Dr. Cook and assistants have carefully explained to me the nature, goals, limitations, and possible complications of this procedure and alternative forms of treatment. I had the opportunity to ask questions about the procedure, its limitations, and possible complications.

All items contained herein apply to these procedure(s):
1. Cook Weekend Alternative to the Facelift™
2. _____
3. _____

I clearly understand and accept the following:
1. The potential benefits of the proposed procedure(s).
2. The possible alternate medical procedure(s).
3. The probability of success.
4. The reasonable anticipated consequences if the procedure(s) are not performed.
5. The possibility that additional services/fees may be required, including, but not limited to, anesthesia, laboratory, medications, and/or surgical facility or hospital use.
6. The goal of cosmetic surgery is improvement, not perfection. Satisfaction is based on realistic expectations. No one should expect that the procedure will remove all excess skin, all excess fat, or every wrinkle, or smooth and tighten skin perfectly. It does not guarantee the reduction of any measurements or weight.
7. The average time off from work and social activities is usually 2–3 days, but in some patients this may be extended.
8. The final result may not be apparent for 3–6 months postoperatively.
9. Occasionally, to achieve the best possible result, additional procedures may be required. There will be a charge for any additional operation performed.
10. Strict adherence to postoperative instructions is necessary in order to achieve the best possible results.
11. The surgical fee is paid for the operation itself and subsequent postoperative visits.
12. I will not drive for 24 hours after the procedure.
13. I give my permission for the administration of anesthesia, as deemed appropriate by the physician.
14. Protective eye covering will be provided to protect my eyes from accidental laser exposure. Accidental exposure to laser is extremely rare but possible.

continued

TABLE 4-2 Continued

Although complications following surgery are infrequent, I understand that the following may occur:

1. Bleeding is rare. In rare instances it could require hospitalization and blood transfusion. It is possible that blood clots or fluid may form requiring surgical drainage or medication.
2. Swelling, crusting, skin irregularities, lumpiness, hardness, and dimpling may occur postoperatively. Most of these problems will disappear with time and massage, but they may persist permanently.
3. If loose skin is present in the treated areas, it may or may not shrink to conform to the new contour. In rare cases wrinkling may persist.
4. Infection is rare, but should it occur, treatment with antibiotics and/or surgical drainage may be required.
5. Possible numbness or increased sensitivity of the skin over treated areas may persist for months, and in rare cases may be permanent.
6. Objectionable bruising and scarring are rare but possible, and may result in discoloration or texture changes of the skin. This is usually temporary but may rarely be permanent. To minimize the chances of this, I understand that it is important for me to follow all preoperative and after-care instructions carefully.
7. Dizziness may occur following surgery, particularly upon rising from a lying or sitting position. If dizziness occurs, exercise caution while walking and do not attempt to drive a car.
8. As the dermal resurfacing heals and the skin redrapes itself, in rare instances the skin may appear more wrinkled and the neck may feel tighter. In almost all cases this resolves, but in rare instances it may persist.
9. Allergic or toxic responses to anesthesia are extremely rare, but possible.
10. In addition to these possible complications, I am aware of the general risks inherent in all surgical procedures and administration of anesthetic.
11. (For chin implant procedures only.) Rare but possible complications include: extrusion (pushing out of the implant), malposition (abnormal location of the implant), bone absorption, hypesthesia of the lip (full or partial loss of sensation), and allergies. These complications may require removal of the implant.

My signature certifies that I have discussed the above material thoroughly with Dr. Cook and assistants. I understand the goals, limitations, and possible complications of the above procedure(s). I wish to proceed with the operation. I authorize and direct Dr. Cook and/or associates or assistants of his choice to perform these procedures on me and/or to do any other additional therapeutic procedure that his judgment may dictate to be advisable, reasonable, or necessary for my well-being.

Patient signature: _____ Date _____
Witness signature: _____ Date _____
Physician signature: _____ Date _____

TABLE 4-3 PATIENT CONSENT FORM FOR PHOTOGRAPHY

I hereby agree that photographs/video tapes may be taken of _____ by Dr. Cook. I agree that these photographs/videotapes may be used in any manner as part of educational, medical, and promotional programs developed on behalf of Dr. Cook.

Exclusions, if any: _____
Patient signature: _____ Date _____
Patient printed name: _____
Witness signature: _____ Date _____
Witness printed name: _____

TABLE 4-4 MEDICAL HISTORY

Name of patient: _____

Name and address of your family doctor: _____

May we contact your doctor in regard to any medical problem that may arise?

Are you considered a healthy person?

Are you now taking ANY drugs or medications? Which ones and how often?

Are you allergic to ANY medications? Which ones?

Have you ever received local anesthesia (Novocain or Xylocaine) from a dentist or doctor?

Have you ever received general anesthesia?

Have you ever had any bad reaction to either local or general anesthesia? Please describe.

_____

Do you take blood thinners? Which ones?

Do you take vitamins regularly? Which ones?

Do you take aspirin products or anti-inflammatory medicines or headache medicines? Which ones?

Do you have permanent makeup? What areas?

List all previous surgeries, peels, and dates: _____

Have you had (please circle):
    malignant hyperthermia
    fever blisters (herpes simplex)
    heart trouble
    blood pressure related problems
    liver problems, gallbladder problems, or yellow jaundice
    kidney disease
    diabetes
    stomach problems, indigestion, or ulcers
    bleeding tendency or excessive bruising
    any part of your body paralyzed or numb
    psychiatric consultation
    epilepsy—convulsions or seizures
    broken bones of the face, neck, jaw, or back
    back trouble
    abnormal chest x-rays
    abnormal electrocardiogram (ECG)
    asthma or other respiratory problems
    any medical treatment for nervous condition
    excessive scarring or abnormal healing. Explain _____
    tuberculosis
    thyroid problems
    any other illness. If so, please list: _____

Do any family members have:
    heart trouble
    excessive scarring
    diabetes
    asthma
    excessive bruising
    bad reaction to anesthesia
    tuberculosis
    high blood pressure
    psychiatric or "nerve" problems
    thyroid problems
    excessive bleeding tendency
    malignant hyperthermia

continued

TABLE 4-4 Continued

Do you:
    wear contact lenses?
    have dentures, false teeth, caps, or bridges?
    smoke? How much?
    drink alcohol? How much?
    have any loose teeth or gum disease?
    object to blood transfusions?
    think you are pregnant? Date of last menstrual period: _____
    have any contagious or infectious conditions? Which ones? _____

TABLE 4-5 PATIENT INFORMATION SHEET—MEDICATIONS

Be sure you have completed the medical history form which we gave to you, and advise us of any allergies you have. PLEASE TELL US IF YOU ARE ALLERGIC TO ANY OF THE MEDICATIONS ON THIS SHEET.

1. Chlorhexidine gluconate (Hibiclens) cleanser
    You may purchase this without a prescription. Take two showers and wash your hair, face, and body with this cleanser, once the night before and once the morning of surgery. Do not get this cleanser in your eyes.
2. Phytonadione (Mephyton; vitamin K) 5 mg
    Take 1 tablet twice a day for 2 weeks, starting 1 week before surgery. Do not take Mephyton if you have a history of blood clots or thrombophlebitis.
3. Cefadroxil (Duricef, 500 mg; or other antibiotic and dosage as appropriate)
    Take 1 capsule twice a day for 7 days, starting the day before surgery.
4. Acetaminophen (Tylenol)
    Take 2 tablets 3 times a day as needed for discomfort.
5. Diazepam (Valium)
    The nurse will supply you with tablets when you leave the office on the day of surgery. You will receive written instructions explaining how to take them. It is essential that you take the medication as specified.
6. Oxycodone hydrochloride and acetominophen (Percocet)
    Take 1 tablet every 3–4 hours only if you need it for discomfort following surgery.
7. No aspirin, aspirin-containing products, ibuprofen, niacin, or vitamin E are to be taken prior to surgery. If you currently take these, stop them immediately. They can cause bruising. Tylenol is the only pain reliever permitted before surgery.

TABLE 4-6 PREOPERATIVE INSTRUCTIONS FOR PATIENTS

1. Please inform our staff of any health problems, previous surgeries, allergies, and any medications that you are taking.
2. DO NOT TAKE ASPIRIN OR IBUPROFEN PRODUCTS OR VITAMIN E PRIOR TO SURGERY, AND FOR 1 WEEK AFTER SURGERY. These products can cause bleeding. These include aspirin (Empirin), ibuprofen (Nuprin, Motrin, Advil), naproxen sodium (Aleve, Anaprox), naproxen (Naprosyn), piroxicam (Feldene), vitamin E, any other anti-inflammatory medicine, arthritis medicines, vitamins, and cold/flu medications. Call our nurse if you have any questions. The only pain medication allowed prior to your surgery is acetaminophen (Tylenol).
3. Be sure that you take all medications as directed.
4. Please advise our staff of any removable dental appliances or contact lenses. Please do not wear contact lenses the day of surgery.
5. Please do not wear any jewelry or bring any valuables such as purse, wallet, or watch on the day of your surgery. We cannot be responsible for any lost items.

continued

TABLE 4-6 Continued

6. DO NOT CONSUME ANY ALCOHOLIC BEVERAGES FOR SEVERAL DAYS PRIOR TO SURGERY AND 1 WEEK AFTER SURGERY. Alcohol may cause bleeding and may interfere with the other medications you are taking.
7. Arrange for a responsible adult to bring you to and from the office, NOT A TAXI DRIVER OR YOURSELF. DO NOT PLAN TO DRIVE A VEHICLE FOR 24 HOURS.
8. Arrange for a friend to stay with you for the first night after your surgery.
9. Take 2 showers, one the night before surgery and one before surgery. Wash your hair and face with Hibiclens™ cleanser (may be purchased at the drug store). DO NOT GET THIS IN YOUR EYES. You may apply conditioner to your hair, but do not use hair spray or mousse.
10. Eat a light meal the morning of surgery. NO CAFFEINE OR ALCOHOL. Limit your fluid intake on the morning of surgery to 1 glass.
11. (FOR FACIAL SURGERY ONLY.) Purchase 4 bags of frozen peas to use as cold compresses after surgery.

YOUR SURGERY HAS BEEN SCHEDULED FOR (date): _____

PLEASE REPORT TO THE OFFICE AT (time): _____

TABLE 4-7 POSTOPERATIVE INSTRUCTIONS FOLLOWING BODY LIPOSCULPTURE

▸ Swelling and discoloration may be present following liposculpture surgery. The amount varies from person to person. Careful attention to these postoperative instructions will help to minimize your discomfort after surgery.
▸ Please keep in mind that results from liposculpture surgery take time. You may not see your final results for 6 weeks to 6 months.
▸ You must have an adult friend drive you to and from the office on the day of surgery and stay with you for the first 24 hours. You may not leave the office in a taxi.
▸ Plan to rest in bed the remainder of the day of surgery. You may walk at a normal pace, but do not engage in any strenuous activity. You may resume your normal daily activities after 24 hours.
▸ You will have drainage from the incision sites for the first 24–48 hours. This is normal; it is the extra tumescent anesthetic solution used during surgery. The drainage will be much less after the first 48 hours but a small amount can continue for the first week.
▸ You must drink at least 1 glass of water every hour until 11 P.M. the night of surgery. Continue drinking 4–6 glasses water each day, in addition to other fluids of your choice. No alcohol, tea, coffee, or carbonated drinks should be consumed for at least 3 days after surgery. Do not drink sport drinks (Gatorade), vegetable juice (V8), tomato juice, or other high salt drinks, as salt will cause swelling.
▸ You must eat a small meal as soon as you arrive home after your surgery. Choose foods that are low in salt (to help prevent swelling). A well-balanced diet is important in achieving good results from your surgery. Foods that cause gas, such as beans and broccoli, should be avoided.
▸ No alcoholic beverages are allowed for 1 week before and several days after the surgery, or for as long as you are taking antibiotics or pain medication.
▸ You will be discharged wearing a surgical compression garment. Wear this garment 23 hours a day for the first week. In the following weeks, wear it 12–23 hours a day depending on your needs.
▸ The morning after surgery, remove the garment and take a shower. Shower with soap and water, and wash the incision sites with Hibiclens cleanser. Put on a clean surgical garment over the pads.
▸ After 2 days, continue cleansing with Hibiclens but do not use the absorbent dressing. The incisions will heal better if they are uncovered and dry.
▸ You may resume normal daily activities after 24 hours. Returning to work depends on the type of work you do, your age, and the amount of liposculpture surgery you had. Most people return to work 1–2 days after surgery.

continued

TABLE 4-7 Continued

▸ The morning after surgery, you should take a 2–3 mile walk. This is very important to relieve swelling. Continue walking and other mild physical exercise in the days following surgery. Your physical status, age, and the amount of surgery done will determine when you may resume heavy activity.

▸ You will be given various medications to take. Keep a written record of the times medications are taken. Take all medications as prescribed; do not skip or double up on medications. See the separate medication sheet for a list of medicines to take and to avoid.

▸ Pain is usually minimal and easily controlled by medication. Do not take aspirin or nonsteroidal anti-inflammatory medication prior to surgery; you may take only acetaminophen (Tylenol). After surgery, you may take naproxen sodium (Anaprox), oxycodone hydrochloride and acetominophen (Percocet), etc. Do not drive if you are taking Percocet.

▸ Swelling and fluid retention are possible after this type of surgery. Drinking plenty of water will act as a natural diuretic to reduce swelling.

▸ Do not drive on the day of surgery. After the first day, you may drive if you are not taking Percocet or other medications that cause drowsiness.

▸ Avoid water immersion until your incisions have completely healed and the scabs have fallen off. This includes a tub bath, swimming pool, or Jacuzzi.

▸ Protect yourself from the sun. The incision sites may darken if they receive too much sun.

▸ Do not use self-tanning creams until bruising has resolved.

▸ Feel free to call our office at any time, day or night, if you have questions or problems.

TABLE 4-8 POSTOPERATIVE INSTRUCTIONS FOLLOWING FACIAL SURGERY

▸ Swelling may be present following facial surgery. This is usually minimal and temporary, but varies from person to person. Careful attention to these postoperative instructions will help to minimize any swelling, discoloration, and discomfort after surgery.

▸ You must have an adult friend drive you to and from the office on the day of surgery and stay with you for the first night. You may not leave the office in a taxi.

▸ Plan to rest in bed the remainder of the day of surgery, to help prevent bruising and swelling.

▸ Elevate your head at all times. Sleep on 2 pillows for 1 week. This will help to prevent swelling.

▸ Apply cold packs to your face for the first 8 hours after surgery until bedtime, alternating 15 minutes "on" and 15 minutes "off." This will reduce bruising and swelling. Bags of frozen peas or soft ice packs are excellent for this purpose. Purchase four such packs so you can keep two in the freezer while using the other two. Do not put ice cubes directly on your skin; just gently lay the cold packs on your face. Remember to keep the operative area and tapes dry.

▸ For the first 48 hours after surgery, confine your activities to resting and gentle activities that do not elevate your heart rate or blood pressure. If you are receiving a chin implant, avoid contact sports for 2–3 weeks.

▸ Be gentle to your face and neck, and avoid trauma to the area.

▸ Tapes will be applied to your face and neck postoperatively. Do not remove these tapes. They will be removed at your follow-up office appointment. Keep them dry.

▸ If you have sutures on your neck, they will be removed 2–3 weeks after surgery. The sutures are clear and very unobtrusive.

▸ You will be given a chin strap to wear after surgery. Wearing this strap helps to prevent bruising, decreases swelling, and gives your neck a better shape.

▸ You may shower or bathe in lukewarm water, but keep your neck tapes dry. After we remove the tapes, you should wash your neck incision sites twice a day for 1 week. Wash with soap and water, then hydrogen peroxide, and then apply antibiotic ointment. Do not use adhesive bandages (Band-Aids) in this area.

▸ You will be given various medications to take. Keep a written record of the times medications are taken. Take all medications as prescribed; do not skip or double up on medications. Do not take aspirin or other nonsteroidal anti-inflammatory medications for 10 days after surgery. See the separate medication sheet for a list of medicines to take and to avoid.

▸ Do not drive on the day of surgery.

continued

TABLE 4-8 Continued

- ▸ If at any point in your recovery you experience swelling, resume the application of cold packs to the area.
- ▸ Avoid sunburn of your face and neck. Wear a hat and protect yourself from the sun. The incision sites may darken if they receive too much sun.
- ▸ Do not use self-tanning creams for 2 weeks following surgery.
- ▸ Feel free to call our office at any time, day or night, if you have questions or problems.

TABLE 4-9 PATIENT SELF-CHECK LIST BEFORE SURGICAL PROCEDURE

Please assist us by making sure the following items are completed before surgery.

Items to be accomplished at your preoperative appointment:

1. We have given you written instructions.
2. We have taken your pictures.
3. You have read your instructions and discussed them with us.
4. You have given us your medical history.
5. You have received your prescriptions.
6. You have received your laboratory request forms.
7. You have signed all consent forms.
8. You have paid for your surgery in full.

Items to be accomplished before your surgery date:

1. You have obtained your laboratory work. Try to obtain this 4 weeks prior to your surgery date.
2. Your primary care physician has sent us a letter, stating your medical history, medications, approval for cosmetic surgery, and other requested information.
3. You have made arrangements for someone to stay with you for 24 hours after surgery.
4. You have arranged for someone to bring you to the office the day of surgery and to take you home. You will need to be accompanied home by a responsible adult. Please give us the name of this person.
5. You have given us the telephone numbers where you can be reached the day before surgery, the day of surgery, and the day after surgery.
6. You have purchased all items on the medication list we have given you. You may need to start some medications up to 1 week in advance of surgery.
7. You should stop taking aspirin, anti-inflammatory products, and vitamin E, 7 days before surgery.
8. (For body liposculpture only.) You will be provided with a surgical garment by this office. We will also suggest alternative garments you may want to purchase 1 week after surgery.

▷ Physical Examination

The patient is weighed and a brief physical examination is performed. A medical history is obtained, with an emphasis on allergies, medications, and previous surgical experience.

We prefer that all patients, if possible, be Class I or Class II surgical risks, even though the procedure that we plan to do is under local anesthesia with sedation. If they are Class II, careful consideration is given to their underlying medical condition and its possible effect on the surgery and subsequent recovery. An ECG may be obtained when indicated, and is preferred for patients over 60 years of age. We request that all patients have a clearance letter from their primary physician.

Laboratory Studies

Currently, we order the following laboratory tests: complete blood count (CBC), complete chemistry panel, coagulation profile, hepatitis screen, and urinalysis. If possible, we like to receive these results up to 2 weeks prior to the surgical procedure so that if any abnormalities are noted, additional testing or appropriate action can be taken.

Generally speaking, the results of laboratory findings in our patient population tend to fall within normal ranges. The most common finding requiring action is prolonged bleeding time. In most cases this is caused by the patient taking aspirin-containing products or certain types of anti-inflammatory medications, which they are advised to stop. Patients who have a mild iron-deficiency type anemia can be started on iron at this time. If the urinalysis shows a sign of urinary tract infection, appropriate antibiotics are instituted. Any other abnormalities in the laboratory studies should be handled with the patient on an individual basis.

In California, all patients are offered the opportunity to predonate autologous blood so that they may have it on hand during the procedure, if necessary. However, in the thousands of liposculpture procedures we have performed, we have never found it necessary to transfuse any patient.

Medications

The patient is placed on appropriate prophylactic antibiotics, generally starting the day before surgery and continuing for 7 days. We prefer cefadroxil (Duricef), 500 mg b.i.d., in patients who are not sensitive to penicillin. If they are allergic to penicillin, we order other appropriate antibiotics.

If not contraindicated, patients are also placed on vitamin K (Mephyton), 5 mg b.i.d., for the week prior to and the week following surgery. In our experience, this helps reduce the amount of postoperative bruising. Some patients may not tolerate vitamin K and may complain of nausea and/or headaches; in this case, the medication should be discontinued.

In patients who are very anxious about having surgery, a mild relaxing medication such as diazepam (Valium), 5 mg, may be prescribed to take at bedtime and/or on the morning of the surgery.

Any medications that the patient takes on a regular basis are reviewed, and any that may conflict with those to be taken preoperatively or given during surgery should be discontinued, if possible. If necessary, the patient's primary care physician or specialist may be contacted to discuss a particular medication.

Patients are instructed not to take any medications containing aspirin, ibuprofen, niacin, vitamin E, or similar substances prior to surgery, and not to drink alcoholic beverages. Patients are instructed to wash with an antibacterial soap such as chlorhexidine gluconate (Hibiclens) the night before surgery as well as the morning of surgery, avoiding their eyes.

▷ Photography

Next, the patient is taken to a special photography area (Fig. 4-1). Preoperative photographs are taken from multiple angles that clearly show the areas to be treated, as well as the adjacent sites. If possible, it is best to do all photography in the same location, so that when the postoperative photographs are taken, the lighting, distances, and proportions will be the same for easy comparison. Photographs should be developed and printed as soon as possible, so that they will be available on the day of surgery.

Patients may be photographed in bikini-type swimsuits for women and brief swimsuits for men. These suits permit a clear view in the photographs, and also make it possible to give copies of the photographs to the patient to compare with their subsequent results. However, some physicians photograph their patients without clothes. Photographs provide a permanent visual record of the patient's preoperative condition and are useful to the surgeon during the surgery. Also, the photographs help to show patients the changes that have occurred.

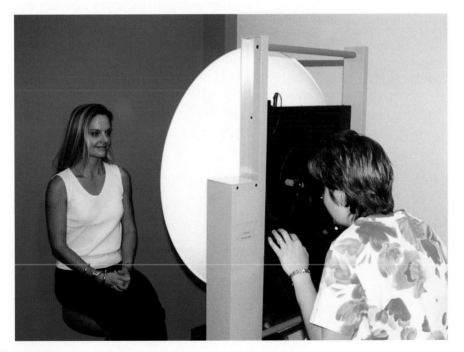

Figure 4-1
Preoperative photography of a facial surgery patient.

▷ Surgical Garment

At this visit, we determine what type of surgical garment the patient will need, arrange to order it, and give instructions for its use. A good surgical garment should give adequate compression to the area of surgery and adjacent sites to help speed recovery, as well as providing a good comfort zone for the patient. We usually order two identical garments so that the patient can wear one while washing the other.

The period of time that the patient actually wears the garment will vary. We usually recommend body garments be worn almost full time for up to 1 week, and thereafter approximately half time for as long as the patient feels that it is providing support and comfort. Obviously, the thicker the fat pad is, the longer the patient may want to wear the garment. Most patients understand the benefits of this type of garment, and patient compliance as to usage is excellent.

▷ Final Review

After the various tasks outlined here have been completed, we like to have a final review with patients, giving them an opportunity to ask any questions and outlining realistic expectations. We confirm that patients have been given prescriptions, laboratory order sheets, and pre- and postoperative care instructions, as well as copies of all the other paperwork that has been discussed with them. Patients are encouraged to call with any other questions or points that they may need to have further clarified.

CHAPTER 5

TUMESCENT ANESTHESIA

Goals of Tumescent Anesthesia ▶ *Use of Tumescent Solution* ▶ *Formulating the Tumescent Solution* ▶ *Preinfiltration Anesthesia* ▶ *Lidocaine Dosage Limit* ▶ *Lidocaine Levels and Toxicity* ▶ *Checklist for Tumescent Anesthesia*

In 1987, dermatologist Jeffrey Klein described the tumescent technique for liposuction, in which large volumes of physiologic saline solution containing very dilute concentrations of lidocaine and epinephrine are injected into the subcutaneous fat. Enough fluid is infiltrated to make the tissues swollen and firm, hence the name "tumescent." This technique was proven to be consistently safe and effective when properly performed (1—3). The composition, concentration, and total amount of tumescent fluid infused are absolutely critical to a successful result.

Tumescent anesthesia allows liposuction to be performed under local anesthesia over larger areas than previously possible, without the need for general anesthesia or intravenous sedation and without lidocaine toxicity. The tumescent technique uses direct infiltration of a saline-based or similar solution to deliver lidocaine, epinephrine, and other medications into the subcutaneous area.

The presence of very dilute epinephrine, in the range of 1:1,000,000, causes vasoconstriction in the subcutaneous fat. This in turn has three important consequences: bleeding during and after the procedure is greatly decreased; the local anesthetic effects of the lidocaine are prolonged; and the systemic absorption of lidocaine is delayed, permitting larger doses to be administered than could be safely done without the epinephrine.

The vasoconstriction caused by dilute epinephrine in the tumescent solution produces a hemostasis that is widespread and profound. As a result, the quantity of blood lost during the aspiration procedure is very small. Only 12 mL of blood are lost for each liter of pure fat that is extracted during tumescent liposuction, with approximately 1% of the aspirated material being whole blood (4). This virtual elimination of blood loss during the tumescent liposculpture procedure has eliminated the need for blood replacement therapy for patients undergoing tumescent liposculpture. In my practice, I have never transfused a patient.

The tumescent anesthesia produced by very dilute lidocaine (generally, 0.05% or 0.1%) permits liposculpture to be performed totally under local anesthesia. This anesthesia is sufficient for an extended surgical procedure. In the thousands of cases I have performed under tumescent local anesthesia, I have never had to abandon a procedure because of patient intolerance to the suctioning. The residual effect of the anesthesia allows patients to be free of any significant discomfort for at least the first 10 to 16 hours after surgery, and in many cases for as long as 24 hours after surgery.

I recommend tumescent technique as the desirable way to perform liposculpture. It was developed to minimize the risk of the surgery and to optimize patient comfort. When properly performed, it provides a safe way to perform larger volume liposuction, while virtually eliminating the risks associated with intravenous or general anesthesia. This technique also allows a variety of cannulas to be used to achieve optimal results.

I do all my procedures under tumescent anesthesia only, using no intravenous or inhalational anesthesia. I give sedation intramuscularly and sublingually to the extent necessary to maintain the patient's comfort. This method of delivering limited sedation has proven to be adequate, safe, and easy to administer and monitor, and it is well tolerated by patients.

Some physicians elect to use a modified tumescent technique by combining tumescent anesthesia with general or intravenous anesthesia. However, this method may be more dangerous than tumescent anesthesia alone. In some cases, the combined method has resulted in serious complications. The increased risk may stem from the inherent risks of general and intravenous anesthesia. Maintenance of fluid balance can also be a problem. If tumescent solution has been infiltrated, the volume of fluid given intravenously should be held to a minimum, just enough to maintain the IV.

The tumescent solution can be administered either by the surgeon or by an experienced infiltration specialist, such as an anesthesiologist or registered nurse. Use of ancillary personnel helps to reduce fatigue to the surgeon and allows more effective utilization of his or her time for the liposculpture procedure itself.

▷ Goals of Tumescent Anesthesia

When the surgeon decides to use tumescent anesthesia, he or she will have a number of goals in mind, including, but not limited to:

- ▶ Targeting the effects of drugs in local tissue areas
- ▶ Maximizing the concentration of drugs locally
- ▶ Delaying the systemic absorption of drugs
- ▶ Extending the time of action of local drugs

> ▶ Decreasing systemic drug toxicity
> ▶ Increasing the upper limit of safety for total dosage
> ▶ Use of hydrostatic dissection for tissue expansion
> ▶ Avoiding the need to use intravenous or general anesthesia
> ▶ Increasing the safety of liposuction procedures
> ▶ Minimizing blood loss during the procedure

▷ Use of Tumescent Solution

It is very important to be precise in the formulation and administration of tumescent solution. Any deviation from a fixed protocol can lead to severe surgical complications. Every member of the staff, from the surgeon to the ancillary personnel, must be aware of the importance of precise formulation and labeling, consistent handling, and proper record keeping with regard to tumescent solution.

In planning the surgery, one must carefully calculate the amount of lidocaine that will be infused.

At the time of the writing of this book, the actual safe maximum concentration of lidocaine has not been precisely determined. The current estimated maximum dosage of lidocaine for a tumescent liposculpture procedure is 60 mg/kg of body weight. In relatively thin patients, a better safety margin would be 50 mg/kg. These relative values have been determined in clinical evaluations by numerous liposuction surgeons. One must remember that there is no absolute maximum. It is always better to use the least amount of lidocaine possible in each case.

If the patient is thin, so that the permissible amount of lidocaine is reduced, one can infiltrate all areas initially using the 0.05% concentration of lidocaine. Then, in more fibrous areas where typically a higher concentration is required, a relatively small amount of 0.1% lidocaine solution can be infiltrated just prior to suctioning the area. This will achieve good anesthesia while still maintaining a safe limit for total lidocaine administration. One must check for other drug interactions that might additionally reduce the permissible maximum dosage of lidocaine.

Table 5-1 shows a worksheet that can be used to develop an infusion plan. Tables 5-2 to 5-4 show typical calculations for body liposculpture procedures performed under local anesthesia.

All of the initial infiltration is performed according to plan prior to commencing the surgery. This allows careful control of the total amount of lidocaine being infiltrated. The total amount infused at the start of surgery should be less than 60 mg/kg, to allow for additional infiltration during the case.

Throughout the procedure, a staff member should be assigned to accurately document the total dosage of lidocaine administered in milligrams, keeping in mind the estimated maximum dosage in milligrams calculated for that patient's body weight. Medicolegal considerations and the standard of care require that this be done correctly and accurately, to protect the surgeon and the patient.

For best results, tumescent solution is usually made up fresh on the day it will be used. The efficiency of tumescent solution is less than maximal if it is mixed

TABLE 5-1 INTRAOPERATIVE WORKSHEET FOR BODY LIPOSCULPTURE

Date of surgery: _____

Patient's name: _____ Chart #: _____

Patient's weight: _____ pounds

     weight × 2.2 = _____ kilograms

Weight in kg × 60 mg/kg = _____ mg lidocaine maximum

Areas being treated: (circle)

Upper abdomen	Lateral thighs	Buttocks	Breast/Chest
Lower abdomen	Posterior thighs	Calves/Ankles	Lipoma, site: _____
Lateral flanks	Medial thighs	Axillary folds	Other: _____
Posterior flanks	Anterior thighs	Arms	_____
Infrascapular	Knees	Dowager's hump	

Tumescent solution infusion record:

    _____ bags of 0.1% lidocaine used × 1,000 mg = _____ mg

    _____ bags of 0.05% lidocaine used × 500 mg = _____ mg

                Total lidocaine infused: _____ mg

Aspirate record:

    _____ mL of supernatant fat

    _____ mL of infranatant solution

    _____ total aspirate

Cannulas used (circle)

Klein	10 gauge,	12 gauge,	14 gauge	
Capistrano	12 gauge,	14 gauge,	16 gauge	
Pinto	3 mm,	3.5 mm,	4 mm	
Cook	9 gauge,	11 gauge,	3 mm,	3.5 mm
Other:	_____			

TABLE 5-2 TYPICAL INFUSION PLAN FOR TUMESCENT LIPOSCULPTURE OF THE ABDOMEN, FLANKS, AND WAIST

Female patient, 130 lbs. = 60 kg

Maximum allowable infusion of lidocaine
    based on 60 mg/kg of lidocaine maximum
      60 kg × 60 mg/kg = 3,600 mg

Body area	Volume of 0.1% lidocaine (1,000 mg/L)		Volume of 0.05% lidocaine (500 mg/L)	
Abdomen	1,000 mL		500 mL	
Lateral flanks			1,000 mL	
Posterior flanks			500 mL	
Infrascapular			500 mL	
Total lidocaine	1,000 mg	+	1,250 mg	= 2,250 mg

TABLE 5-3 TYPICAL INFUSION PLAN FOR TUMESCENT LIPOSCULPTURE OF THE CHEST, ABDOMEN, AND FLANKS

Male patient, 175 lbs. = 80 kg

Maximum allowable infusion of lidocaine
   based on 60 mg/kg of lidocaine maximum
     80 kg × 60 mg/kg = 4,800 mg

Body area	Volume of 0.1% lidocaine (1,000 mg/L)		Volume of 0.05% lidocaine (500 mg/L)	
Chest	500 mL			
Upper abdomen	750 mL			
Lower abdomen	750 mL			
Lateral flanks			1,000 mL	
Posterior flanks			500 mL	
Infrascapular			500 mL	
Total lidocaine	2,000 mg	+	1,000 mg	= 3,000 mg

several days in advance of surgery. Variables such as pH, temperature, and the concentration of other solutes will vary the shelf life. The vasoconstrictive properties of epinephrine are not stable at a pH ≥ 5. Also, there is a greater risk the lidocaine may precipitate from an older solution or from a solution with a higher pH. In my practice, epinephrine is added just before using the specific 1000-mL volume of saline, to which the lidocaine and bicarbonate have already been added.

    I prefer to warm the tumescent solution to 39 to 40°C before infusion. This reduces stinging during infusion and also helps to minimize patient heat loss during the procedure.

TABLE 5-4 TYPICAL INFUSION PLAN FOR TUMESCENT LIPOSCULPTURE OF THE ANTERIOR THIGHS, MEDIAL THIGHS, AND KNEES

Female patient, 130 lbs. = 60 kg

Maximum allowable infusion of lidocaine
   based on 60 mg/kg of lidocaine maximum
     60 kg × 60 mg/kg = 3,600 mg

Body area	Volume of 0.1% lidocaine (1,000 mg/L)		Volume of 0.05% lidocaine (500 mg/L)	
Anterior thighs			2,000 mL	
Medial thighs	750 mL			
Knees	250 mL			
Total lidocaine	1,000 mg	+	1,000 mg	= 2,000 mg

▷ Formulating the Tumescent Solution

I use two concentrations of tumescent solution, made up fresh on a daily basis. In addition to lidocaine (0.1% or 0.05%) and epinephrine (1:1,000,000), the solutions contain sodium bicarbonate and triamcinolone acetonide (Kenalog). The sodium bicarbonate serves as a buffer. The triamcinolone may help to reduce postoperative swelling and induration; at this time, it is an optional addition to the tumescent solution.

The 0.1% lidocaine solution contains:

- ▶ Lidocaine, 1,000 mg/L (0.1% concentration)
- ▶ Epinephrine, 1 mg/L (1:1,000,000 concentration)
- ▶ Sodium bicarbonate $NaHCO_3$, 10 mEq/L
- ▶ Triamcinolone acetonide (Kenalog), 10 mg/L

and is made up as follows:

1,000 mL of normal saline solution (0.9%) in an infusion bag
10 mL of 8.4% sodium bicarbonate $NaHCO_3$ (1 mEq/mL)
50 mL of 2% lidocaine
1 mL of 0.1% epinephrine (1:1,000) added just before infusion
1 mL of triamcinolone acetonide (Kenalog), in the form of a 10 mg/mL
    suspension, added with the epinephrine just before infusion

The 0.05% lidocaine solution contains:

- ▶ Lidocaine, 500 mg/L (0.05% concentration)
- ▶ Epinephrine, 1 mg/L (1:1,000,000 concentration)
- ▶ Sodium bicarbonate $NaHCO_3$, 10 mEq/L
- ▶ Triamcinolone acetonide (Kenalog), 10 mg/L

and is made up as follows:

1,000 mL of normal saline solution (0.9%) in an infusion bag
10 mL of 8.4% sodium bicarbonate $NaHCO_3$ (1 mEq/mL)
25 mL of 2% lidocaine
1 mL of 0.1% epinephrine (1:1,000) added just before infusion
1 mL of triamcinolone acetonide (Kenalog), in the form of a 10 mg/mL
    suspension, added with the epinephrine just before infusion

The sodium bicarbonate and lidocaine may be added to the infusion bag up to approximately 24 hours in advance of surgery. A syringe containing the epinephrine and triamcinolone acetonide (Kenalog) is taped to the outside of the bag, to be injected just prior to infusion (Fig. 5-1).

It is vitally important that each bag be labeled with its exact contents, along with the date it was made up and the initials of the person who made it (Fig. 5-2).

Just before infusing, warm the infusion bag to approximately 39 to 40°C in a microwave oven. The temperature can be checked by holding a thermometer

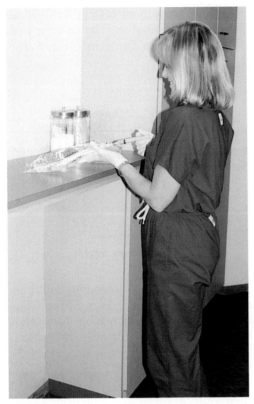

Figure 5-1
Mixing tumescent solution on the day of surgery.

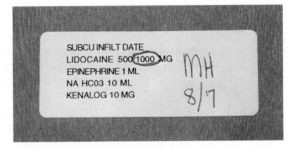

Figure 5-2
Label placed on bag of tumescent solution.

against the bag. Staff will quickly learn the length of time needed to reach this temperature, which tends to be consistent for a given microwave oven.

▷ Preinfiltration Anesthesia

Preliminary anesthesia of each infiltration site is obtained by injecting a small bleb of a commercially prepared local anesthetic mixture containing 2% lidocaine and 1:100,000 epinephrine. It is important that this anesthetic mixture be stored in a separate cabinet from the reagents that will be used to mix up the tumescent solution.

▷ Lidocaine Dosage Limit

Before beginning the infusion, a plan should be devised showing how much tumescent solution is to be infiltrated into each body area. This plan should indicate the total amount of lidocaine in milligrams that will be infused. It should aim for less than the estimated maximum allowable amount of 60 mg/kg of body weight, so that additional tumescent solution may be used to "top off" the anesthesia during surgery. Typical presurgical calculations are shown in Tables 5-2, 5-3, and 5-4.

▷ Lidocaine Levels and Toxicity

The surgeon should be familiar with the signs of lidocaine toxicity, which are a function of lidocaine peak plasma concentration. Toxicity may result from the following factors:

- ▶ Overdose
- ▶ Excessively rapid systemic uptake
- ▶ Impaired hepatic metabolism
- ▶ Drug interactions

To help prevent toxicity, the total dosage of lidocaine that will be infiltrated should be calculated. Because lidocaine is metabolized by the liver, hepatic function should be checked as part of the preoperative laboratory testing. All medications that the patient is taking should be reviewed for possible drug interactions. The tumescent formulation should be followed carefully. It is very important that the epinephrine be added to each 1000 mL of solution that is prepared, because epinephrine slows the absorption of lidocaine.

The following table shows the toxicity effects that can result from various plasma lidocaine concentrations:

3–6 μg/mL	Subjective signs: lightheadedness, euphoria, paresthesias, restlessness, drowsiness
5–9 μg/mL	Objective signs: nausea, vomiting, tremors, blurred vision, tinnitus, confusion, excitement, psychosis, muscle fasciculations
8–12 μg/mL	Seizures, cardiac depression
12 μg/mL	Coma
20 μg/mL	Respiratory arrest
26 μg/mL	Cardiac arrest

▷ Checklist for Tumescent Anesthesia

- ▶ Make up tumescent solution fresh on a daily basis.
- ▶ Allow only experienced staff to formulate the solutions.
- ▶ Label each bag carefully with its exact contents.
- ▶ Have only two formulations of lidocaine in the formulary, to reduce the possibility of an error in dosage.
- ▶ Plan carefully the concentration and total amount of lidocaine that will be infiltrated, in a particular area and in the total procedure.

▶ Use lidocaine (Xylocaine) only; do not substitute any other related local anesthetic. Especially, do not use bupivacaine, which may be cardiotoxic in large doses and make it difficult to resuscitate.

▶ Keep in mind the estimated maximum recommended lidocaine dosage for tumescent procedures: 60 mg/kg, in general, and possibly reduced to 50 mg/kg in relatively thin patients.

▶ When specifying and calculating dosage, use milligrams, rather than volume amounts or percentages.

▶ Accurately document the total dosage of lidocaine administered throughout the procedure in total.

▶ Warm the tumescent solution to 39 to 40°C before infusion.

▶ As a control, save all used infiltration bags so as to keep an accurate running total of the amount of lidocaine that has been infiltrated.

▶ Infuse solution with a rotary infusion pump.

▶ Begin infiltration with a 21-gauge spinal needle to reduce tenderness, and then utilize a 14-gauge multipore infusion cannula.

▶ Keep incision sites as small as possible, preferably 1.0 to 2.5 mm.

▶ Do not suture the incision sites, to allow good drainage of all areas.

REFERENCES

1. Bernstein G, Hanke W. Safety of liposuction: a review of 9478 cases performed by dermatologists. *J Dermatol Surg Oncol* 1988;14:1112–1114.
2. Hanke CW, Bernstein G, Bullock S. Safety of tumescent liposuction in 15,336 patients. *Dermatol Surg* 1995;21:459–462.
3. Hanke CW, Lee MW, Bernstein G. The safety of dermatologic liposuction surgery. *Dermatol Clin* 1990;8:563–568.
4. Klein JA. Tumescent technique for local anesthesia improves safety in large-volume liposuction. *Plast Reconstr Surg* 1993;92:1085–1098.

CHAPTER 6

ULTRASONIC LIPOSCULPTURE

Internal Versus External Ultrasound ▶
Intraoperative External Ultrasonic Liposculpture ▶
Postoperative External Ultrasound

For many years, external ultrasound has been used safely as a diagnostic and therapeutic tool for a variety of conditions. One of its well-established uses is as a treatment for postoperative swelling after liposculpture. I have used it for this purpose since approximately 1990 (1). I found that postoperative treatment with external ultrasound decreases swelling and discomfort and promotes rapid healing. It is high in patient satisfaction and is also very safe when properly performed.

A more recent development has been the application of external ultrasound before or during the tumescent liposculpture procedure itself. External ultrasound can make the procedure easier for the surgeon, and it can also decrease postoperative bruising, swelling, and discomfort for the patient. When properly used by trained personnel, it is very safe.

Internal and external applications of ultrasound have been tried in conjunction with tumescent liposculpture. However, there have been many problems associated with internal ultrasound. I currently use only external applications.

As the technology improves, internal ultrasound may yet fulfill its promise as an adjunct to tumescent liposculpture. The principles discussed here for the use of external ultrasound would apply to internal-ultrasound-assisted procedures as well. The ultrasonic cannula would only be used for the first few minutes of the procedure in any area, to soften and prepare the tissue. Liposculpture would then be completed using conventional methods.

Before using ultrasonic energy for this or any purpose, the physician should be knowledgeable about its usage and side effects, as well as possible complications. Any additional personnel using this modality should also be adequately trained.

▷ Internal Versus External Ultrasound

In recent years, there has been a renewed interest in the use of ultrasonic technology to enhance the procedures of liposculpture. The technology has evolved, and several types of ultrasonic liposculpture have been developed. One technique uses external ultrasound, where the sound energy is applied through a transducer held against the body. Another, called internal ultrasound, involves special surgical instruments and cannulas that generate sonic energy and apply suction.

Ultrasound is believed to affect adipose cells via several mechanisms: thermally, micromechanically, and through the phenomenon of cavitation. Internal ultrasonic liposuction utilizes the principles of cavitation. The exact mechanism by which external ultrasound affects the tissues is currently not clear.

The internal application of ultrasound requires a fluid medium to conduct the ultrasonic waves. Because tumescent liposculpture by its very definition has a fluid medium, the internal ultrasound technique seemed ideal for use with tumescent liposculpture procedures. However, the internal ultrasonic technique has not yet lived up to its potential.

Early methods of internal ultrasonic liposuction have been abandoned by most of the European surgical community because of numerous complications. Newer ultrasonic units have been introduced in the United States and have proven with time to be somewhat safer. However, internal ultrasound is still associated with many complications and problems. In some cases these have included perforation of the abdominal cavity, burning of incision sites and overlying skin, seromas, poor cosmetic results, and a variety of other complications.

Another problem with internal ultrasonic liposuction is that it depends on the use of special cannulas. Therefore, the surgeon cannot use most of his or her existing cannulas during a procedure involving internal ultrasound.

I have used internal ultrasonic liposculpture in my practice, but I found it unsatisfactory. Results were no better than with my standard tumescent liposculpture technique. I decided to avoid the so-called "hot probe" tipped cannulas because of the safety issues that have been reported. I elected to use water-cooled versions of the internal ultrasonic cannula, but I found these cannulas technically difficult and very time consuming to use.

Therefore, at the time of this writing, I will discuss only the use of external ultrasonic energy to improve the results of liposculpture. As the technology improves, internal ultrasound will presumably become a viable option for a properly trained surgeon.

▷ Intraoperative External Ultrasonic Liposculpture

After the patient has been prepared and the tumescent solution infiltrated (as described in Chapter 7), external ultrasound is applied to all areas to be treated. The only exception, in my practice, is that I do not use ultrasound on a very thin neck.

I use a Rich-Mar external ultrasound unit (Bernsco or Byron Medical, see Appendix) (Fig. 6-1). Energy is applied to body areas at 3 W/cm^2, and to lower face

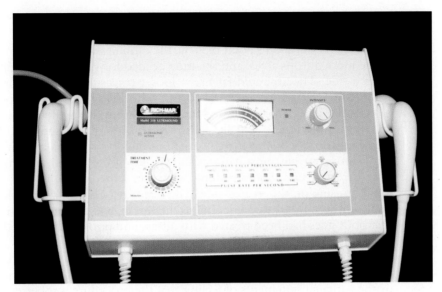

Figure 6-1
Rich-Mar ultrasound unit.

and neck areas at 1 W/cm^2, continuous wave, at 1 MHz. The external transducer, which measures 10 cm in diameter for the body and 5 cm in diameter for the neck, is moved slowly and continuously in a circular fashion over the areas to be treated for 10 to 15 minutes per body area (Fig. 6-2). Sterile ultrasonic gel is used to improve the conduction between the transducer and the patient. Moderate pressure is applied to thicker fatty areas. Care must be taken to avoid bony areas. The probe should never be applied at this wattage to nontumesced areas and should never be applied in a static manner.

When the ultrasound treatment is completed and the tumescent solution has been "topped off" (see Chapter 7), liposculpture is performed in the usual manner.

I studied the effect of preoperative external ultrasound in a series of 30 patients (1). External ultrasound was administered preoperatively on one side of the body and not the other. The surgeon was not told which side had been treated. The surgeon and the nursing staff made comparative observations. On their post-

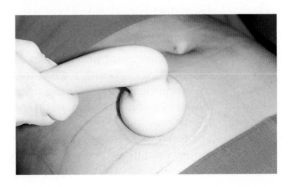

Figure 6-2
Applying ultrasound before liposculpture.

operative visits, patients gave their subjective observations of swelling, bruising, and discomfort, comparing the treated and untreated sides.

From the surgeon's point of view, the cannulas were easier to move, especially in the more fibrous areas, and the time needed for surgery was slightly less on the treated side. The aspirated fat had a looser consistency and a more milky white color, compared to the aspirated fat from the areas that were not pretreated with ultrasound. The temperature of the tissue during liposculpture was monitored, and it was found to be actually slightly lower after ultrasound treatment. This decrease is probably due to the constriction of blood vessels after tumescence.

Postoperatively, most patients showed less bruising and swelling on the ultrasound treated side. Some patients were the same on both sides; none showed more bruising on the treated side. The majority of patients noted less discomfort on the ultrasound treated side. In fact, many patients commented that they wished that both sides had been treated with ultrasound prior to the procedure. No complications were noted.

The cosmetic results of sculpting in the treated areas were comparable to those on the side that was not pretreated with ultrasound. I was most impressed by the patients' statements of feeling that the procedure was better for them. The nursing staff also noted improvements, which were consistently reproducible in patients. I have continued to perform external ultrasound during tumescent liposculpture procedures with very favorable results.

▷ Postoperative External Ultrasound

I have used external ultrasound in my practice since approximately 1990 to treat postoperative liposculpture patients. I have found that external ultrasound decreases swelling and discomfort, promotes rapid healing, and is not only high in patient satisfaction but also very safe when properly performed, with no complications noted.

When using ultrasonic energy postoperatively, I utilize 0.5 W/cm^2 for the face and neck areas, and 1.0 W/cm^2 for the body areas. If the area is significantly indurated, I usually inject the site with triamcinolone (Kenalog), 2 mg/mL, injecting 2 to 5 mL per body area. Then I treat each site with ultrasound for 5 to 10 minutes. This procedure is performed once a week until the swelling and/or discomfort is resolved. Many patients experience a decrease in symptomatology and swelling immediately on completion of the ultrasound treatment, even before leaving the office.

The same principles apply as for the intraoperative use of external ultrasound (as described previously). The probe should never be in a static position. It should be constantly in motion using a gentle, slow, circular rotation. Clear ultrasonic gel is used as a conductive medium for the ultrasonic waves.

Although I do not use postoperative ultrasound in all patients, it is an excellent technique for patients who experience postoperative discomfort or swelling, and significantly expedites their recovery.

REFERENCE

1. Cook WR Jr. Utilizing external ultrasonic energy to improve the results of tumescent liposculpture. *Dermatol Surg* 1997;23:1207–1211.

CHAPTER 7

SURGICAL PROCEDURE FOR TUMESCENT LIPOSCULPTURE

Day of Surgery ▶ *Marking the Skin* ▶ *Incision Sites* ▶ *Heparin Lock* ▶ *Intraoperative Monitoring* ▶ *Sedation* ▶ *Infusion of the Tumescent Anesthetic Solution* ▶ *Intraoperative Pretreatment With Ultrasound* ▶ *Liposculpture Procedure* ▶ *Endpoint* ▶ *Closure*

▷ Day of Surgery

Patients are greeted by the nurse in charge of their case and taken back to the preparation area. At this time, a final review of the planned procedure, alternatives, and risks is carried out. Patients should confirm their understanding of the areas to be treated. Only those sites that have been previously agreed on in writing, on a signed consent form by the patient, will be treated. Any last-minute changes to this plan must be in writing and must be initialed by the patient before being given any sedative medications.

A preoperative physical examination is performed, including the patient's orientation, heart, lungs, and vital signs. The patient's medications are reviewed one last time. The areas to be treated and adjacent sites are now scrubbed with povidone-iodine (Betadine) or, if the patient is allergic to iodine, with a solution such as chlorhexidine gluconate (Hibiclens).

▷ Marking the Skin

With the patient in the standing position, the areas to be treated, landmarks, and incision sites are carefully marked with a gentian violet marking pen. I use a gentian violet marker because it will not tattoo the skin through any of the incision sites. Other permanent markers may have their dye leach into the opening used for the liposculpture and correspondingly tattoo the site.

Marking is done while the patient is standing up, so that the physician can easily visualize the desired results. When those same areas are under the influence of expansion with tumescent solution and various positional changes, the markings take on a very important role in achieving optimal surgical results.

Patients can interact in this marking process and point out areas that are disturbing to them, and the surgeon can again review the anticipated results. This is a good time to indicate areas that are less likely to improve, and areas that will probably not be affected by the surgery. If there are areas of asymmetry, this is noted in the marking, and patients are reminded that although attempts will be made to correct these asymmetries, some side-to-side differences might persist.

Each surgeon will develop his or her own system of markings to indicate elevations, depressions, old surgical scars, or any other areas to treat or avoid treating during the course of the surgery. My personal system of markings for the different anatomic areas and the incision sites will be shown in the appropriate chapters. Each mark should have some significance to the surgeon.

In some areas, a circular outline of the fatty deposits is helpful (Fig. 7-1). In other areas, long linear marks are useful to indicate the relative path that will be taken by the cannula. These can be especially important in elongated areas such as the thighs, where there are few anatomical landmarks to help the surgeon attain maximum uniformity in suctioning. These long markings will also show the de-

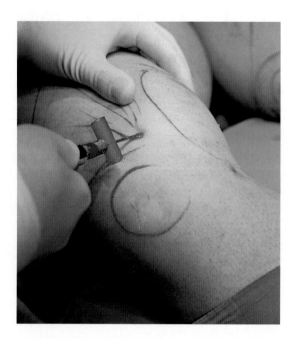

Figure 7-1

Incisions and markings for the knee and anterior thigh. The surgeon is suctioning the medial knee fat pad.

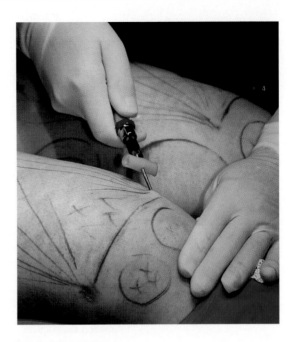

Figure 7-2

Incisions and markings for the knee and anterior thigh. The surgeon is suctioning the infrapatellar fat pad.

gree of crisscrossing that will be achieved from the different incision sites (Fig. 7-2).

I use a circle within a circle, as on a topographical map, to show areas of depression. It is important to be aware of areas that are normally depressed, or possibly surgically depressed due to previous liposuction procedures, so that the adjacent sites can be blended in to achieve good contouring.

Also, points of attachment that the surgeon does not want to violate should be marked, for example, the infragluteal crease and the inframammary crease. Ultimately, whatever system of marking the surgeon selects, he or she should be consistent in using these markings so that they are meaningful to the surgeon and to the nursing staff that is assisting on the case.

▷ Incision Sites

When considering the proper placement of incision sites for the best results, the following three approaches may be used: minimal, moderate, and multiple. The minimal approach allows for the least amount of crisscrossing with the cannula. The moderate approach is defined as scattered, permitting crisscrossing. Finally, the multiple approach calls for incision sites approximately every 4 inches.

For best results, I recommend a moderate number of incision sites. The advantages of a moderate approach include adequate crisscrossing; ability to utilize a variety of cannula sizes and lengths; adequate access to "difficult to reach" areas, such as the waist; limited number of sites to heal; and most importantly, high patient satisfaction.

In choosing the incision sites, one should be sure that there is a drainage site at the most inferior aspect of the anatomic areas treated.

TABLE 7-1 CRASH CART EMERGENCY SUPPLIES

A Drawer
  Airway supplies
    3 oral airways
    3 nasal airways
    5 tubes of lubricating jelly
    1 bite stick
    1 suction syringe
    1 nasal cannula
    1 oxygen mask, simple
    1 oxygen mask, reservoir
    1 pair of goggles
  IV supplies
    4 IV start kits
    8 IV catheters: 18G, 20G, 22G
    4 butterfly
    1 microdrip tubing
    1 macrodrip tubing
    1 normal saline, 500 mL
    1 Ringer's lactate, 500 mL
    1 pair of goggles
  Intubation supplies
    1 laryngoscope handle, with batteries
    2 laryngectomy blades, 1 straight, 1 curved
    4 endotracheal tubes: 6, 7, 8
    3 syringe, 10 mL
    1 stylet
    1 Magill forceps
    1 Toomey syringe
    1 NG tube
    1 suction tube with Yankauer
    1 minitrach/cric kit
    1 whistle tip suction catheter
    1 pair of goggles
B Drawer
    1 Ringer's lactate, 500 mL
    1 normal saline, 500 mL
    2 D5W, 250 mL
    1 macrodrip tubing, 15 drop
    1 microdrip tubing, 60 drop
C Drawer
    2 adenosine (Adenocard), 6 mg/2 mL, 3-mL syringes
    2 atropine 1-mg preload
    2 bretylium 500 mg, 10-mL syringes
    3 epinephrine, 1:10,000 preload
    3 lidocaine, 100-mg preload
    1 lidocaine 2-mg drip
    1 microdrip tubing, 60 drop
    1 nitroglycerine, 0.4 mg
    2 nifedipine (Procardia), 10 mg
    2 verapamil hydrochloride, 5 mg, 3-mL syringes

continued

TABLE 7-1 Continued

D Drawer
 3 epinephrine (adrenalin), 1 mg, 1-mL syringes
 2 diphenhydramine hydrochloride (Benadryl), 50-mg preload
 1 dextrose, 25-g preload
 1 albuterol (Proventil)-inhaler
 2 furosemide (Lasix), 40-mg preload
 1 naloxone hydrochloride (Narcan), 0.4 mg/ml, 10-mL syringe
 1 flumazenil (Romazicon), 1 mg, 10-mL syringe
 1 steroid (Decadron), 3-mL syringe
E Drawer
 1 BP cuff
 3 ECG stickies
 1 tube defib gel
 8 syringes, variety
 1 stethoscope
 tape, 2×2 gauze squares, adhesive bandages (Band-Aids)

▷ Heparin Lock

With the patient in the supine position, a heparin lock is inserted. This is purely a safety precaution and is utilized only when medications or fluids must be given intravenously. In the majority of cases it is not necessary to use the heparin lock, but it is a good safety tool to have available. My patients almost never require any intravenous fluids because the tumescent solution used during the case provides an adequate amount of hydration. I do not administer any sedation by means of the intravenous route. Rarely, if a patient develops nausea, intravenous medication such as prochlorperazine (Compazine) may be given.

▷ Intraoperative Monitoring

Patients are monitored throughout the procedure as to their pulse, ECG, O_2 saturation, and blood pressure. Also, patients are administered low-flow oxygen, approximately 2 L/min. An emergency crash cart should be available in the operating suite and be fully equipped with the standard medications that would be used for resuscitation. A typical list of medications and supplies for an emergency cart is shown in Table 7-1. All crash-cart supplies and their expiration dates should be checked on a regular schedule, after which the cabinet should be secured with an easily breakable plastic band, indicating that the medications are all present and accounted for.

▷ Sedation

After the patient is prepared and draped, markings in place, and monitors and oxygen apparatus attached, sedation is administered, either intramuscularly or sublingually. It is important to determine the patient's allergic status and not to administer any medications where there may be a question of allergy in the past. For initial sedation, I generally select midazolam (Versed), either 2.5 or 5 mg intramuscularly, depending on the patient's age and body weight, as well as meperidine (Demerol), 50 to 100 mg intramuscularly, and hydroxyzine (Vistaril), 25 to 50 mg intramuscularly. These medications have proven very safe and very easy to monitor, and they give the patient additional comfort, especially during the infiltration phase of the procedure, when the tumescent solution is being infused into the subcutaneous area.

For many patients, this initial dosage of intramuscular sedation is all that is required, because once the tumescent anesthetic solution is in place, liposculpture can proceed with very little discomfort. Depending on the number of areas that are being treated and the patient's sensitivity, additional Versed and Demerol may be given during the surgery, if necessary. This is especially helpful during long contouring procedures.

If necessary, diazepam (Valium) may also be given sublingually, 5 mg approximately every hour. This not only provides some mild sedation, but also provides excellent control of the shivering that occurs in some patients. The shivering is probably due to the vasoconstrictor effect of the epinephrine in the tumescent solution, which can cause a cooling effect on the skin. I always have my patients wear a warm surgical cap and wool socks during surgery, which helps to reduce the cold feeling they may experience.

▷ Infusion of the Tumescent Anesthetic Solution

All the incision sites should have been marked previously with the patient in a standing position. Generally, the tumescent solution is infiltrated through these incision sites. Each incision site is first infiltrated with a solution of 2% lidocaine (Xylocaine) and 1:100,000 epinephrine, in the form of a small bleb. Using this stronger concentration provides complete anesthesia for the incision sites and also produces an initially greater degree of vasoconstriction to avoid capillary ooze, which may occur even around the smallest of skin openings.

After the area has been anesthetized in this way, the incision is made either with a no. 11 surgical blade or with a 16-gauge Nokor needle (Becton Dickinson & Co., Rutherford, N.J.), attempting to limit the incision site to approximately 1 mm on the face or 2 mm on the body. If at some point a larger incision is needed, I use intraoperative tissue expansion, stretching the body incision to 3 mm with curved iris scissors.

Infiltration is then begun with the appropriate concentration of tumescent solution. See Chapter 5 for a discussion of the principles, safety considerations, dosages, and mixing of the tumescent solution.

The tumescent solution is warmed to 39 to 40°C. This can be done in a microwave oven or in a water bath. Warming of the solution helps to reduce the patient's heat loss during surgery. Also, the tumescent solution has fewer tendencies to sting and burn during the infiltration phase if it is warmed.

The infiltration is begun using a mechanical infiltration pump and a 21-gauge spinal needle (Figs. 7-3, 7-4). This is an excellent tool for the initial phase of the

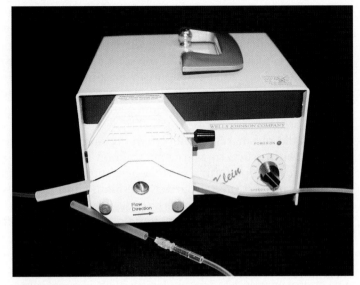

Figure 7-3
Infiltration machine for tumescent liposculpture.

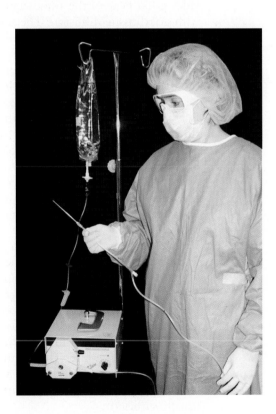

Figure 7-4
Tumescent solution infiltration machine and a
spinal needle, prior to infiltration of tumescent solution.

infiltration because it produces minimal discomfort and yet delivers an adequate amount of tumescent solution. The solution is infiltrated in a spokelike radial fashion around the incision site. The needle is moved forward and backward in a gentle to-and-fro motion, advancing the rotation approximately 1 cm each pass, until the maximum radial distribution possible has been infiltrated. Then the infiltrator should move to each incision site in turn and perform the same type of spoke–wheel distribution of the tumescent solution. If it is necessary to infiltrate a distant area that cannot be reached by way of an incision site, one can take the spinal needle and make a small bleb in the subdermal plexus area from within the subcutaneous tissues, so as to achieve good anesthesia for re-entry through the skin surface, then perform a spoke–wheel approach at the site of the bleb.

In this manner, in a progressive fashion, all of the areas are given what one might consider a preanesthesia dose of solution. This can be done with little or no discomfort to the patient. A very low flow rate is required for this initial infiltration. The rotary infusion pump that we utilize is set on one of the lower settings on the variable speed dial.

After this initial phase, the infiltrator switches to a 14-gauge infiltration cannula approximately 12 inches in length. This is essentially a long tube with multiple openings near the end, which produces a sprinkling effect of the solution into the tissues. This cannula is very effective because it has a small diameter but provides good flow of the tumescent solution, infiltrating from all sides of the port with good tissue diffusion. The speed of the infusion pump is now increased.

The amount of tumescent solution to be infiltrated in each area will vary according to many factors. The overriding factor to keep in mind is the total amount of lidocaine that may be safely infiltrated into the patient. This should be planned out prior to the surgery, with a clear understanding of the factors limiting the total amount of solution that can be utilized. Infusion of each section must stay carefully within the predetermined limits, which have been set with regard to the estimated maximum amount of solution that can be utilized for the entire procedure. (See Chapter 5 for a complete discussion of this aspect of the surgery.)

After the sites appear to be well tumesced and are clinically anesthetic, it is helpful to wait for at least 15 to 20 minutes in order to allow the solution to diffuse into the tissues. Since the anesthesia is long lasting, a much longer waiting time can be used if desired. At this point external ultrasound can be applied, if indicated.

On beginning the surgery, a final infiltration of the area is done to confirm that the area is adequately anesthetized, as well as to "top off" the solution. Only a small amount of tumescent solution is usually required for this final infiltration. I generally use a 12-inch 12-gauge spatula-type cannula. If this cannula is well tolerated, one can be reasonably certain that surgery can now proceed under local anesthesia with minimal discomfort to the patient.

In all areas, I reinfiltrate with tumescent solution approximately halfway through the procedure. This reinfiltration expands the working space and, consequently, achieves good yield. It also reinforces the anesthesia and augments the vasoconstrictor effect. A small amount of tumescent solution (100 to 200 mL) is usually sufficient.

Written records should be kept of the amount of tumescent solution infiltrated, and the empty infiltration bags should be retained as a double-check. Table 5-1 shows a possible format for keeping these records.

▷ Intraoperative Pretreatment with Ultrasound

After the tumescent solution has been infiltrated, I pretreat the body areas with external ultrasound, if indicated. In my experience, this pretreatment makes the procedure easier for the surgeon and promotes postoperative comfort and more rapid healing for the patient. (See Chapter 6 for a description of this procedure.) Before using ultrasonic energy in conjunction with liposculpture or any procedure, the practitioner must be adequately trained in the uses, precautions, and possible complications of this technology.

▷ Liposculpture Procedure

Liposculpture surgery calls for a combination of medical knowledge, artistic sense, and visual and tactile interpretation. The surgeon must also have sufficient physical stamina and conditioning to avoid fatigue, so that he or she will be as focused at the end of the procedure as at the start.

Some general considerations apply to sculpting technique in all areas of the body. These include:

▶ Proceed in a uniform, orderly, and organized fashion throughout the body areas.
▶ Pull the cannula in and out in a to-and-fro motion.
▶ Do not randomly sweep an area with the cannula like a windshield wiper.
▶ Transect the fatty layer uniformly in an orderly progression throughout.
▶ Do not repeat strokes in one place to "dig a hole," and then try to match the surrounding areas to the newly created depression.
▶ Suction from the deep to the superficial plane and feather all the surrounding areas.
▶ Keep the tip of the cannula elevated and controlled by the nondominant "smart" hand.
▶ Keep the suction ports facing downward.
▶ Monitor the aspirate in the tube for excess blood.
▶ Keep the vacuum pump on its maximum setting.

In positioning the patient, I often find it helpful to use a pillow, as will be related in subsequent chapters. I have found the optimal pillow to be an 8 × 8 × 30-inch foam cushion with vinyl covering, which of course is covered with a sterile drape during surgery. I use custom-made pillows, but positioning pillows are also available from Bernsco and Wells Johnson (see Appendix).

Please refer to Chapters 9 through 18 for discussions of specific liposculpture techniques for each anatomic area.

▷ Endpoint

To determine when enough fatty tissue has been removed from a particular area requires using a number of criteria. None of these criteria are absolute. Experience gained in performing numerous cases will be the best yardstick for most surgeons. The following guides should help the surgeon to establish when enough is enough.

Remember that overcorrection may be as undesirable as undercorrection. The surgeon should decide on a relative thickness of skin and fat that he or she wants to remain in a particular area based on the relative thickness in adjacent body areas, the patient's overall weight, and the amount that may realistically be removed in one procedure.

The pinch test (Fig. 7-5) can give the surgeon a feel for how much fat is remaining. To perform the pinch test, grasp the skin and subcutaneous layer between the thumb and index finger. The actual thickness of the skin and subcutaneous fat is one-half the thickness of the tissue between the fingers.

A variant of the pinch test is the use of the nondominant hand flat on the patient's skin during suctioning. This permits the surgeon, on an ongoing basis, to

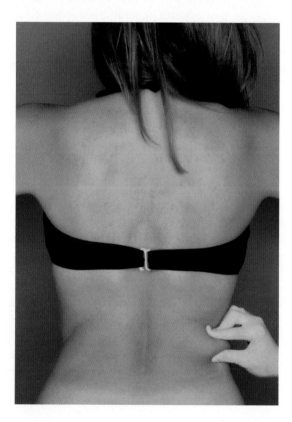

Figure 7-5

The pinch test, showing a thickened posterior flank fat pad.

determine by feel the thickness of the remaining fat pad over the cannula. For this reason, many people have referred to the nondominant hand as the "smart" hand.

The visual appearance of the treated area and the comparison between this and other body areas can also give a good guide to the endpoint. The surgeon desires to remove an optimal amount of fat; however, it is probably better to leave more rather than to remove too much. Removal of an excess amount of fat in one area may leave a too thin appearance and may not balance with adjacent areas. The surgeon should leave an adequate amount of fat overlying the muscle so that the patient achieves a smoother, more natural contour. The desired amount of fat will vary from one body site to another. Remember that fat is what gives the body its shape.

▷ Closure

I do not suture the incisions, but leave them open. In a study that I performed a number of years ago, I left the incision sites open on one side and closed them on the contralateral side. I found that healing was much better on the nonsutured side. Drainage was improved, swelling and ecchymoses were decreased and resolved more quickly, and the incision itself healed more rapidly.

Of course, this advice is contingent on keeping the incisions small during surgery. My goal is to keep all incisions on the body to a size of 2 mm in width. If a slightly larger incision is needed for a particular cannula, I use the intraoperative tissue expansion technique. This consists of placing a pair of curved iris-type scissors in the small opening and expanding the opening so that on completion of the surgery in that site, the incision will shrink back down to its small size for optimal closure during the postoperative period. Also, one must be sure that there is a drainage site at the most inferior aspect of each anatomic area treated.

POSTOPERATIVE PERIOD FOR TUMESCENT LIPOSCULPTURE

Discharge ▶ *After Discharge* ▶ *Postoperative Follow-Up* ▶ *Postoperative Sequelae and Complications*

▷ Discharge

Because liposculpture is performed using only intramuscular sedation and local anesthesia, patients are normally alert at the completion of the procedure. The nursing staff can begin immediately to prepare the patient for discharge.

All the operative sites are cleansed with chlorhexidine gluconate (Hibiclens) solution and dried. A small amount of antibiotic ointment, such as bacitracin, is placed around the incision sites, and an absorbent dressing is placed over the incisions. For the first 24 hours postoperatively, a large amount of fluid discharge can be anticipated from these sites, which are not sutured. I have found that leaving the small incisions open to drain facilitates healing. In side-by-side studies, I noted that the tissue sites where free drainage was allowed had much less swelling and less ecchymosis. Also, the incisions themselves healed more rapidly.

The compression garment is now positioned over the surgical sites. This should be a lightweight garment that provides adequate compression to the areas and is easy to put on and remove. By this time, the patients are usually in a sitting position.

Patients are then moved to the recovery area, where they can rest, take fluids in the form of juices, have a small snack, and visit the restroom. After a suitable period the monitors are discontinued, the heparin lock is removed, and the patient is prepared for discharge.

TABLE 8-1 PATIENT INSTRUCTIONS FOR IMMEDIATE AFTERCARE FOLLOWING BODY LIPOSCULPTURE

READ THESE INSTRUCTIONS IMMEDIATELY FOLLOWING SURGERY

- When you arrive home, set an alarm clock so that you will know when to take your diazepam (Valium). You have been given 2 Valium tablets. You need to take the first Valium tablet at _____ o'clock and the second Valium tablet at _____ o'clock.
- Take your antibiotic and phytonadione (Mephyton) tonight with crackers or other food. Taking them on an empty stomach may cause nausea.
- Rest the remainder of this day. You should have assistance when you get up to use the bathroom, in case you experience dizziness.
- You must drink at least 1 glass of water every hour until 11 p.m. tonight. Continue drinking 4–6 glasses of water each day, in addition to other fluids of your choice. No alcohol, tea, coffee, or carbonated drinks should be consumed for at least 3 days. Do not drink sport drinks (Gatorade), vegetable juice (V8), tomato juice, or other high salt drinks, as salt will cause swelling.
- You must eat a small meal as soon as you arrive home after your surgery. Choose foods that are low in salt (to help prevent swelling).
- You will have drainage from the incision sites for the first 24–48 hours. This drainage is normal; it is the extra tumescent anesthetic solution used during surgery. The drainage will be much less after the first 48 hours, but a small amount can continue for the first week.
- Wear your surgical garment continuously until the morning after surgery. Then you may remove it briefly to shower. Be sure to have someone with you when you remove the garment. Be sure that you are adequately hydrated before removing the garment.
- Shower with soap and water the morning after surgery. Wash the incision sites with chlorhexidine gluconate (Hibiclens). Cover loosely with gauze. Do not use tape or adhesive bandages (Band-Aids), as these can cause irritation. Put on a clean surgical garment over the pads.
- Physical exercise may be started tomorrow. A 2–3 mile walk is strongly encouraged the morning after surgery. Your physical status, age, and the amount of surgery done will determine when you may resume heavy activity.
- You may resume normal daily activities after 24 hours.
- Do not drive the day of surgery.
- You may shower as often as you like, but avoid water immersion until your incisions have completely healed and the scabs have fallen off. This includes a tub bath, swimming pool, or Jacuzzi.

Before leaving the office, the postoperative instructions are reviewed with the patient and the accompanying person. A friend, family member, or private duty nurse must accompany the patient on discharge and should stay with him or her until the next morning. Although patients are given postoperative instructions before surgery (see Tables 4-7, 4-8), I usually give them a separate sheet of instructions for immediate postoperative care at the time of discharge (Tables 8-1, 8-2). This instruction sheet is reviewed with the patient and family members to be sure that they understand the recovery process and can provide the necessary supportive care.

▷ After Discharge

Patients are advised to rest for the remainder of that evening, take additional food as desired, and maintain a good fluid intake. The importance of hydration cannot be overstated to the patient and caregiver. I recommend drinking 1 glass of water

TABLE 8-2 PATIENT INSTRUCTIONS FOR IMMEDIATE AFTERCARE FOLLOWING FACIAL SURGERY

READ THESE INSTRUCTIONS IMMEDIATELY FOLLOWING SURGERY

▸ When you arrive home, set an alarm clock so that you will know when to take your diazepam (Valium). You have been given 2 Valium tablets. You need to take the first Valium tablet at _____ o'clock and the second Valium tablet at _____ o'clock.

▸ Take your antibiotic and phytonadione (Mephyton) tonight with crackers or other food. Taking them on an empty stomach may cause nausea.

▸ Rest in bed the remainder of the day of surgery, to prevent bruising and swelling.

▸ Elevate your head at all times. Sleep on 2 pillows for 1 week. This will help to prevent swelling. You may want to sleep in a recliner or lounge chair.

▸ Apply cold packs to your face for the first 8 hours until bedtime, alternating 15 minutes "on" and 15 minutes "off." This will help prevent swelling. Bags of frozen peas or soft ice packs are excellent for this purpose. Do not put ice cubes directly on your skin; just gently lay the cold packs on your face. Remember to keep the operative area and tapes dry.

▸ You must drink at least 4–6 glasses of water every day in addition to other fluids of your choice. No alcohol for at least 3 days. Do not drink sport drinks (Gatorade), vegetable juice (V8), tomato juice, or other high salt drinks, because salt will cause swelling.

▸ Eat soft foods that are lukewarm in temperature—neither hot nor cold.

▸ Do not remove your face and neck tapes. They will be removed at your follow-up office appointment.

▸ Do not remove your neck strap until tomorrow while you bathe. Wear this strap 23 hours a day for the first 3 days, and then as much as possible for the weeks following.

▸ You may shower or bathe in lukewarm water, but keep your tapes dry. After we remove the tapes, you should wash your neck incision sites twice a day for 1 week. Wash with soap and water, then hydrogen peroxide, and then apply antibiotic ointment. Do not use adhesive bandages (Band-Aids) in this area.

▸ Do not drive the day of surgery.

▸ For the first 48 hours after surgery, confine your activities to resting and gentle activities that do not elevate your heart rate or blood pressure.

▸ Be gentle to your face. Avoid trauma to the area.

▸ Feel free to call our office at any time, day or night, if you have questions or problems.

every hour while awake. Patients are told to avoid alcoholic beverages, carbonated drinks, and high-salt drinks such as Gatorade.

The surgical garment is left on for the remainder of the day and throughout the night. If the absorbent dressing becomes saturated, it should be changed by slipping it out from under the garment and repositioning a dry absorbent dressing. Because of the copious amounts of drainage to be expected after body liposculpture, I recommend that the patient wear an absorbent outer covering.

That evening, the patient is instructed to take additional diazepam (Valium), 5 mg sublingually, at two specified times. This medication is recommended for the majority of patients and helps the patient to rest comfortably.

The morning following body liposculpture, patients will remove the garment and dressings and take a shower. They should have someone to assist them when they remove the garment, because the release of the pressure may cause them to become slightly light-headed. They should be well hydrated prior to removal of the garment.

Patients are advised to shower with chlorhexidine gluconate (Hibiclens soap), which they have purchased preoperatively, for the first several days postoperatively. It is important to stress that no water immersion such as a bath, hot tub, or swimming pool may be permitted during the postoperative period until all the incision sites have completely closed. Patients are allowed to shower as many times a day as they desire.

After showering, dry absorbent dressings are placed over the incision sites, and a fresh surgical garment is put on. I normally provide patients with two garments so that one can be washed and dried while wearing the other. The garment is worn 12 to 23 hours a day for the first postoperative week and, thereafter, 12 hours a day for as long as the patient feels it is providing comfort and support. I usually recommend that the garment for body liposculpture be worn for 2 to 3 weeks, depending on the individual case. Patients may discontinue usage whenever they feel the garment is no longer helpful.

Following the shower and a light meal, and while maintaining good hydration with a large amount of water intake, I recommend that body liposculpture patients take a 2-mile walk on the first postoperative day. This movement gets the patient back to normal activities very quickly. It helps to expedite the drainage of the tumescent solution and also helps to reduce the natural tissue edema that may result if the patient remains sedentary. Almost all patients, regardless of age, have been able to carry out this regimen, which expedites their recovery significantly.

On the second full postoperative day, many patients are able to resume light exercise, such as using a stair-stepper or stationary bicycle. I do not recommend impact-type exercises, such as running or any contact sports, for the first few days postoperatively. This will vary from patient to patient. Many patients are able to play a full round of golf 3 or 4 days after surgery. In this regard, each patient should be evaluated individually, depending on their preoperative condition, age, and prior level of sports activities. Patients who have had facial liposculpture generally resume normal activities the first postoperative day.

▷ Postoperative Follow-up

Frequent telephone contact is maintained during the postoperative period to be sure the patient is doing well and following instructions. Patients who have had facial surgery, such as the Cook Weekend Alternative to the Facelift™, return to the office 1 to 2 days postoperatively. After body liposculpture, the patient usually returns for a follow-up appointment in 1 week.

At the time of the follow-up appointment, body liposculpture patients should be completing the course of prophylactic antibiotics. Patients are advised to continue wound care until the healing is complete, and to progressively increase their activity level until they have resumed a normal exercise program. Again, the importance of reasonable dietary intake is stressed. If it is necessary to lose weight, the immediate postoperative period of 6 to 8 weeks is an ideal time for the patient to attain a given weight goal. During this time more rapid weight loss is possible, so that patients can reach their goals in a shorter period of time, thereby realizing possibly even better results from the surgical procedure.

At the end of 3 months, contouring has been achieved in the majority of patients, although in some patients it may take an additional 6 to 9 months before all the swelling recedes and final contouring is achieved. Postoperative photographs are taken at the appropriate time after surgery (Fig. 8-1).

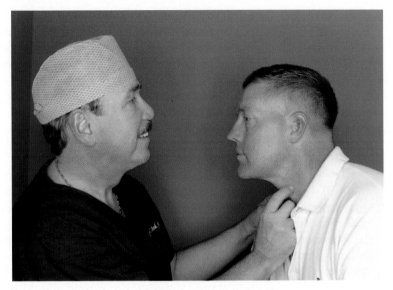

Figure 8-1
Dr. William Cook examines a patient at the 3-week postoperative visit after Cook Weekend Alternative to the Facelift™.

▷ Postoperative Sequelae and Complications

Numerous studies have shown that tumescent liposuction, when performed by properly trained dermatologic surgeons under local anesthesia, is an exceptionally safe procedure that results in only infrequent and minor complications (1–3). A review of 15,336 patients treated by 66 dermatologic surgeons showed no serious complications, such as death, pulmonary embolism, fat embolism, hypovolemic shock, perforation of the peritoneum or thorax, or thrombophlebitis (3). There was no need for transfusions or hospital admissions in this survey group.

In my experience, postoperative complications have been very rare. If good planning has taken place and a set protocol is followed to achieve consistency in surgical procedures, the patient should attain excellent results with minimal to no complications. However, I will describe some possible sequelae and complications, categorized as acute, intermediate, or long-term. A more complete list of possible sequelae and complications is included in the surgical consent forms (Tables 4-1, 4-2).

Acute Sequelae and Complications

Obviously, the patient needs to be monitored during surgery and immediately postoperatively for blood loss. This should be a very rare problem if the surgery is performed properly. In the thousands of surgical procedures I have performed, I have never found a need to transfuse any patient.

Another possible immediate problem is nausea and vomiting, which usually can be eliminated with antiemetic suppositories such as trimethobenzamide HCl (Tigan or Tebamide). One of the most frequent causes of postoperative nausea and vomiting is meperidine hydrochloride (Demerol), so a careful history of intolerance to narcotics should be obtained prior to surgery. I always send the patient home with two antiemetic suppositories and instructions for their use, so that if nausea should develop that evening, it can be treated immediately. In my experience, less than 1% of patients need to use these suppositories.

Another important issue is hydration. Body liposculpture patients need to maintain good hydration, as mentioned previously, drinking 1 glass of water per hour the evening after surgery while awake. If good hydration is not achieved, the patient may feel weak and low on energy. In my experience, patient compliance on this point is generally excellent.

Postoperative pain or discomfort following tumescent procedures is usually minimal. Because the pain threshold of individual patients may vary, I usually give a prescription for oxycodone and acetaminophen (Percocet), to be taken only on an as-needed basis. In my experience, patients rarely need to take this medication. If discomfort is present, it is usually caused by swelling. If the patient becomes ambulatory right away, takes the recommended 2-mile walk the day after surgery, and wears the garment as instructed, swelling is usually minimal.

If the rare infection should develop, the wound should be cultured and appropriate antibiotics prescribed. Surgical intervention is almost never indicated and should be used only if absolutely necessary. In general, good preventive measures as outlined in this book will help ensure that infections do not occur.

Intermediate Sequelae and Complications

Localized edema is uncommon, but is more common in patients who have had previous surgical procedures in the area treated. These may include previous liposculpture, abdominoplasty, or any incisional surgery. Localized edema usually responds well to external ultrasound, as discussed in Chapter 6. It may additionally be reduced by giving the patient triamcinolone (Kenalog), 20 to 40 mg, and betamathosone (Celestone), 6 mg, intramuscularly after surgery.

Any ecchymosis present will usually resolve spontaneously within 10 days to 2 weeks. Bruising tends to be considerably milder than that seen when the procedure is performed under general anesthesia. In my experience, bruising is minimal in body liposculpture patients and nonexistent in 90% of facial surgery patients.

The incision sites should be monitored for the rare instances of hypertrophic healing. If this occurs it can be treated very successfully with intralesional Kenalog, either 2 mg/mL or 5 mg/mL, depending on the patient. A small amount is placed directly into the thickened area. In patients with known histories of keloid formation, as a precaution I inject the incision sites with Kenalog at the completion of the surgical procedure, using a concentration of 2 mg/mL and injecting approximately 0.2 mL into each site.

Hyperpigmentation surrounding the incision sites can be treated with hydroquinone cream or gel, at a concentration of 4%. Higher concentrations may be used if necessary. In my experience, hyperpigmentation is rare. It occurs more frequently in darker skin types and almost always resolves with treatment and sun precautions.

Long-Term Sequelae and Complications

Long-term sequelae and complications are rare in my experience. If the procedure is done correctly, surface irregularities, persistence of excess adipose tissue, or removal of too much adipose tissue should not be a major problem. However, if these should persist after a waiting period of approximately 6 months, an additional smoothing procedure using small cannulas can be attempted. This waiting period is important in order to make sure that the perceived problem was not simply caused by slowly resolving edema in the area. If a secondary treatment is done too soon, the surgeon could very easily over-resect the area, with the resultant defect of a permanent depression in that area. This is an unfortunate cosmetic result and should be avoided. Again, realistic expectations, as well as the goals of the first procedure, must be carefully outlined before attempting a secondary procedure. I very rarely need to perform a secondary liposculpture procedure; this is done in less than one-tenth of 1% of my patients.

Although I rarely see a seroma, if it should occur at any time postoperatively, it can be drained as often as necessary until it is completely resolved, using a 5- to 10-mL syringe with a 18-gauge needle, followed by compression.

REFERENCES

1. Bernstein G, Hanke W. Safety of liposuction: a review of 9478 cases performed by dermatologists. *J Dermatol Surg Oncol* 1988;14:1112–1114.
2. Hanke CW, Bernstein G, Bullock S. Safety of tumescent liposuction in 15,336 patients. *J Dermatol Surg Oncol* 1995;21:459–462.
3. Hanke CW, Lee MW, Bernstein G. The safety of dermatologic liposuction surgery. *Dermatol Clin* 1990;8:563–568.

CHAPTER 9

THE COOK WEEKEND ALTERNATIVE TO THE FACELIFT™: LIPOSCULPTURE OF THE FACE, NECK, AND JOWLS WITH DERMAL LASER RESURFACING

Preoperative Evaluation ▶ *Summary of Surgical Procedure* ▶ *Operative Procedure* ▶ *Postoperative Considerations* ▶ *Results*

Tumescent liposculpture for the face, neck, and jowls is a very effective and safe procedure when properly performed. It is widely done and will improve the appearance of many patients. But in some patients, liposculpture alone is not as effective cosmetically as a rhytidectomy procedure. The cosmetic results in many of these patients can be greatly improved, to the point of being comparable to the results of rhytidectomy, by utilizing an extended tumescent surgical protocol that includes dermal laser resurfacing.

For many years, we have been interested in improving the methods of treating the neck, while avoiding the extensive surgical intervention that a patient is subjected to with traditional rhytidectomy. As partners, we have combined our two specialties and have evolved a combined liposculpture and laser surgical procedure that we call the Cook Weekend Alternative to the Facelift™. This procedure was achieved by pursuing known approved surgical principles, cautiously adding incremental improvements including the surgical laser, and combining them into a format that produces consistent clinical results. This approach uses liposculpture as well as laser resurfacing of the platysma and underside of the dermis, vaporization of subcutaneous fat, resection of a small ellipse of excess submental skin, separation of the neck septae, and plication of the platysma, with or without chin augmentation. Using laser technology, the surgical procedures can be performed under tumescent local anesthesia at the same time as the liposculpture.

The Cook Weekend Alternative to the Facelift™ can lead to significantly superior results with minimal incisions, rare to no complications, and very rapid recovery. Instead of needing weeks to recover from a rhytidectomy, the average patient can undergo our procedure literally "over the weekend," with surgery on Thursday or Friday and a return to work the following week.

This extended procedure creates a natural-looking cosmetic improvement that is far superior to that which can be achieved with liposculpture alone and, in many cases, is comparable to the results achieved by rhytidectomy procedures. Sagging or fatty neck areas are transformed by superior sculpting, good tightening of the neck, significant reduction in skin laxity, and good reduction of the platysmal bands. After this procedure, patients with round and heavy appearing faces gain a thinner, more attractive look. The cheekbones are more prominent, the mandible is more sharply defined, and facial features are in better balance.

In this chapter, we will describe the ten-step, laser-enhanced procedure that constitutes the Cook Weekend Alternative to the Facelift™. This is the procedure we currently use on most face and neck patients. Surgeons who wish to perform simple liposculpture alone can perform steps 1 and 5, omitting the other surgical procedures that utilize a pulsed CO_2 laser and a tissue dissector.

▷ Preoperative Evaluation

Liposculpture may be indicated to correct lipodystrophic changes of the lower face and neck, including "turkey neck" and "double chin." The Cook Weekend Alternative to the Facelift™ is especially useful for patients who display poor cervicomental angles, lax platysma, and in many cases lax skin. However, the technique will not help a person whose skin is severely inelastic beyond repair. Some individuals with poor elasticity in the skin of the face and neck may be helped by first performing either a chemical peel or laser skin resurfacing, and then they can be evaluated for the Cook Weekend Alternative to the Facelift™.

As with any liposculpture procedure, careful consultation and evaluation of the patient is necessary with regard to clinical findings, goals, and realistic expectations on the surgeon's and the patient's part. Patients need to understand that although significant improvement is seen within days, the final results will not be achieved until 2 to 3 months postoperatively. We have noted that patients continue to improve even at 12 months after the procedure.

Changes in the face, neck, and jowls can occur at any age, but generally become more pronounced with aging. We have performed facial liposculpture on all ages from 15 to 75. Patients at the younger end of the spectrum generally desire correction of a genetic pattern of fullness of the neck and face and perhaps a recessive chin, which in many cases was also present in the grandparents and parents. Although these changes can be present in the teens and 20s, most patients do not begin to demonstrate significant changes in the appearance of their face and neck until approximately age 35. At that time the submental fat pad becomes more prominent, the platysma muscle is weaker, and the skin begins to lose its elasticity. By the age of 45 a frank double chin may be present. The skin has lost more of its elasticity, the jowls become thickened and begin to sag, and in many cases the eyelids begin to droop and the skin surface to wrinkle. At age 55, the eyelids may be heavy with many lines, skin folds are deeper, and jowls are sagging more. A turkey neck and double chin are present, in many cases with horizontal platysmal bands forming a ringlike configuration around the neck in several folds. In most cases, these effects of time, gravity, heredity, and sun exposure can be helped by the Cook Weekend Alternative to the Facelift™. In certain patients, additional procedures, such as blepharoplasty and laser resurfacing of the skin, may be indicated.

Before planning liposuction, the distribution of the patient's facial adipose layer must be carefully evaluated. It is important to consider the general facial characteristics of that individual and also to evaluate the family history. One must consider whether the principal problem is bulging of excessive fat or lax skin and muscles. In particular, the turkey neck deformity needs to be evaluated as to its fat content versus the component of the platysma muscle. Sagging jowls may be caused by excess fat or a hypertrophic masseter muscle. Enlarged submandibular glands should be noted and pointed out to the patient. The position of the larynx and hyoid bone should also be considered, and the bony structure of the face needs to be considered. One should also consider whether the cervicomental angle might be improved by inserting a chin implant and suctioning the ptotic chin pad.

In addition to the direct examination, clinical evaluation may be aided by the use of photographs and/or computer imaging. It is important that the angle of the head and position of the camera be in a consistent, specified position. Ideal head angle in the profile view can be achieved by aligning the patient and the camera along the Frankfurt horizontal line, which connects the lowest orbital rim point with the highest point of the ear canal meatus. Many authors have defined various profile lines and proportions. The "general profile line," which is defined as a line that drops from the soft tissue glabella to the soft tissue projection of the chin, may be related to the Frankfurt horizontal. This simple utilization of horizontal and vertical lines can be especially helpful to the surgeon in assessing the need for possible chin augmentation. In anthropomorphic studies of North Americans by Farkas and colleagues (1), the general profile line was found to deviate from the "ideal" zero-degree position an average of minus 4.9 degrees in women and minus 4.7 degrees in men. In studies of facial attractiveness (2), the average general profile line was found to be minus 3 degrees in attractive women and minus 2.7 degrees in the most attractive women studied. As the general profile line approached a more upright posture, the attractiveness of the female profile increased.

When assessing the patient for a chin implant, no firm rules apply as to the size of the implant; these guidelines may be helpful. The most important consideration is not to overcorrect the patient so as to produce too drastic a clinical change in appearance. We use Silastic silicone-rubber implants, which are commercially available in various sizes and shapes (see Appendix). This material is biocompatible with the existing soft tissue and it stimulates the development of a fibrous connective tissue capsule that abuts the implant surface. The Silastic implants are very inert and resist changes in local conditions of the tissues. These implants are comfortable for the patient, give a very natural appearance, and are relatively simple to insert. The surgeon needs only to create a pocket of the appropriate dimensions, carefully position and suture the implant, and suture the pocket closed. The submental or external approach for chin augmentation has many advantages, in that it utilizes the same incision as the remainder of the procedure, yet permits the surgeon to accurately carry out the subperiosteal pocket dissection to whatever height is required for the prosthesis. This preserves the integrity of the buccal sulcus and allows the implants to be positioned with less worry of mental nerve injury.

The role of the platysma muscle is of great clinical importance in addressing any changes that have occurred in the appearance of the neck with age. The platysma tends to become more redundant and lax with the aging process, and this contributes to the appearance of bands in the submental area.

▷ Summary of Surgical Procedure

The Cook Weekend Alternative to the Facelift™ is a ten-step technique for tumescent cosmetic surgery to the face, neck, and jowls. The steps may be summarized as follows:

1. Tumescent liposculpture to the lower one-third of the face, the jowls, excess fat in the ptotic chin, and the entire anterior and lateral neck, covering an area from the mandible to the base of the neck and laterally to the anterior border of the sternocleidomastoid muscle. This removes fat and allows redraping of the submental skin.
2. Laser resection of excessive submental skin (only a small ellipse of tissue removed).
3. Complete transsection of septae on the anterior and lateral neck, so that complete redraping occurs.
4. Separation of the insertions of the platysma muscle to the horizontal bands of the neck, which reduces, and in some cases eliminates, horizontal bands of the neck.
5. Tumescent liposculpture of the subplatysmal fat pad.
6. Laser vaporization of remaining fat globules on the platysma and undersurface of the skin of the neck.

7. Laser resurfacing of the fascia of the platysma muscle to produce tightening of the muscle.
8. Laser resurfacing of the underside of the dermis to produce tightening of the skin of the neck.
9. Insertion of a chin implant, when indicated.
10. Plication of the anterior border of the platysma muscle to produce maximal tightening and reduced platysmal bands, followed by closure of the submental incision.

See Chapter 18 for a discussion of principles and precautions in the surgical use of lasers.

▷ Operative Procedure

The patient is marked in the sitting position. The markings should include the lower face, jowls, chin, and neck with incision points clearly marked (Figs. 9-1, 9-2). These include two 1-mm stab incisions in the submental crease, infra-auricular stab incisions, and an incision in the mucosal surface of the lateral aspect of the upper lip. Markings should clearly show the extent of the planned suctioning, any elevations or depressions, the midline of the chin, and underlying bony structures such as the mandible.

Standard tumescent solution (see Chapter 5) with a lidocaine concentration of 0.1% is infiltrated through stab incisions approximately 1 mm in size in the sub-

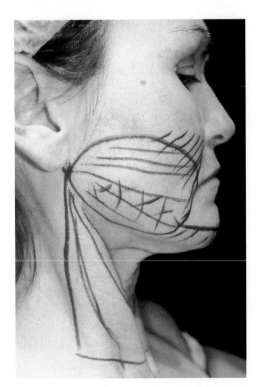

Figure 9-1

Patient marked for Cook Weekend Alternative to the Facelift™. Note infra-auricular incision site.

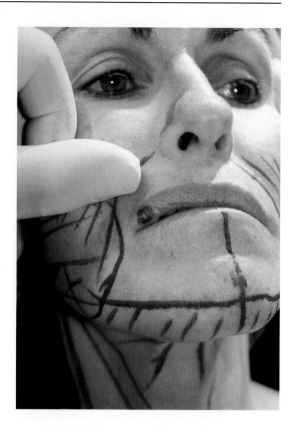

Figure 9-2

Patient marked for Cook Weekend Alternative to the Facelift™. Note markings for mid-chin line incision in the mucosal surface of the lateral aspect of the upper lip.

mental and infra-auricular areas. The entire anterior and lateral neck, jowls, and lower one-third of the face should be infiltrated. The average face and neck will require 500 to 800 mL of fluid to achieve good tumescence for this procedure. If indicated, external ultrasound may be applied at this time (see Chapter 6).

Step 1

After waiting at least 20 minutes to allow good vasoconstriction, tumescent liposculpture is begun (Fig. 9-3). This is done through the submental incision site, using two small stab incisions approximately 1 cm lateral to the midline on each side in the submental fold or the area that will be utilized for the submental incision. In some patients who require a chin implant, the submental incision will be inferior to the submental fold. After the chin implant insertion elevates the submental fold, the incision will still be hidden in the submental area. Having two incisions approximately 2 cm apart permits good crisscrossing during the liposculpture of the neck. It also guarantees the exact line for incision will be maintained, because in many cases the markings may be erased during the suction process and the skin fold that one would normally choose for the incision may disappear due to tumescent expansion of tissues. Using first a 16-gauge and then a 14-gauge Klein spatula cannula, liposuction is performed in the submental region, criss-

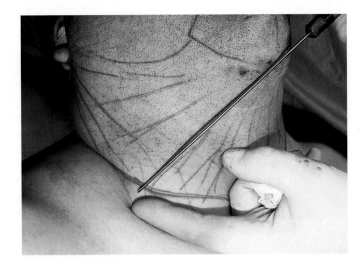

Figure 9-3
Extensive tumescent liposculpture
of the neck and face.

crossing the area and forming the usual honeycomb pattern in the sites of involvement.

After this initial submental suctioning is completed, the infra-auricular incision is used to suction the lower one-third of the face, the jowl area, and the adjacent area of the lateral neck (Fig. 9-4). Usually 16-gauge Klein and Capistrano cannulas are used, making precise passes carefully spaced. This is done in the midplane or deeper to avoid ridging of the cheeks.

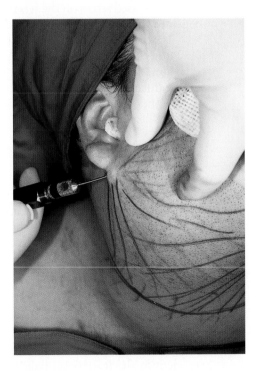

Figure 9-4
Infra-auricular approach to tumescent liposculpture of
the lower one-third of the face and jowl.

The next area of suctioning is through a stab incision approximately 1 mm in size in the mucosal surface of the lateral aspect of the upper lip, approximately 1.5 cm medial to the lateral commisure. I use a 16-gauge Klein spatula cannula and a 16-gauge Capistrano cannula, either 4 or 6 inches in length, to suction the adjacent jowl area and the mound portion lateral to the nasolabial fold, if indicated. I never use larger than a 16-gauge cannula in this area, so that the incision site will close nicely without suturing and leave no apparent cosmetic defect.

After the initial liposculpture is completed, an additional 50 to 100 mL of tumescent solution is infiltrated into the neck region. This infiltration helps to expand the space and provides additional vasoconstriction. The neck region is now sculpted using 14-gauge Klein spatula cannulas, first 4 inches and then 6 inches in length, and finally 12-gauge Klein spatula cannulas, first 4 inches and then 6 inches. During this final sculpting, one should thoroughly cover the areas from the mandibular ridge down to the base of the neck, so that all apparent excess fatty tissue is removed.

Step 2

I now connect the submental incisions with a gentian violet marking pen to outline a 2.5-cm submental ellipse approximately 2 to 3 mm in width. The primary goal of this excision is to provide a working window to allow the surgeon to perform the remaining steps in the procedure. Removal of excess amounts of skin is best avoided, because it may lead to poor wound healing at the incision site due to increased stress on the wound edges. The majority of skin contraction will come from the use of dermal laser resurfacing described subsequently.

See Chapter 17 for a discussion of the surgical use of lasers. I use the Ultra-Pulse 5000 laser (Coherent Medical Group, see Appendix) with initial settings of 15 mJ and 4 W to make the initial skin incision of the ellipse. This "pulsed" mode produces a smaller, usually bloodless incision with minimal tissue damage. I then use the 7-W setting to excise the elliptical piece of skin.

Step 3

A Toledo tissue dissector (Bernsco or Byron Medical, see Appendix) is inserted into this submental incision and is utilized to break all visible septae in the entire anterior and lateral neck. The plane of dissection is important, staying relatively superficial. Adequate hemostasis should be achieved with or without suction cautery using the Valley electrosurgical unit (ValleyLab, see Appendix).

Step 4

The tissue dissector is then utilized to separate the insertion of the platysma muscle into the horizontal bands of the neck. Hemostasis is again controlled with a Valley electrosurgical unit equipped with a special suction cautery tip.

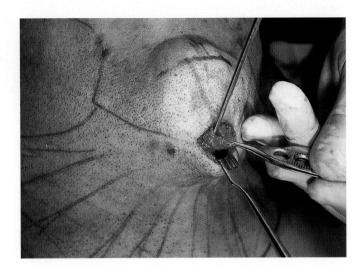

Figure 9-5
Subplatysma fat pad being aspirated under direct vision.

Step 5

Next, I infiltrate the midportion of the platysma muscle with a solution of 2% lidocaine and 1:100,000 epinephrine, approximately 1.5 to 2.0 mL injected into the muscle. This will provide anesthesia and vasoconstriction for the subplatysmal suctioning described subsequently.

A small scissors stab incision is made in the midline of the superior aspect of the platysma muscle. The subplatysmal fat pad is carefully visualized through this small opening and is gently aspirated using a 12-gauge Klein spatula cannula (Fig. 9-5). The fat in this area is very soft, and extreme caution and very slow movements of the cannula are needed, so as not to traumatize any of the adjacent structures. Also, one must carefully monitor the area for good hemostasis following suctioning.

After the subplatysmal pad is removed, direct visualization is made of the jowl areas. Any residual globules of fat in this area are carefully removed, using the same 12-gauge Klein spatula cannula with the openings toward the skin surface.

Step 6

Using the laser, I perform spot vaporization of any persistent fat lobules on the platysma and undersurface of the skin.

Step 7

I then use the UltraPulse 5000 laser in a defocused mode on a 7-W setting to gently resurface approximately 30% of the anterior surface of the platysma muscle, using a crisscrossing randomized pattern. This tightens the fascial surface of the platysma.

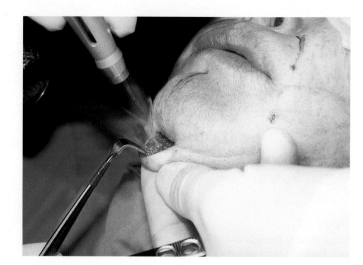

Figure 9-6

Laser resurfacing of the undersurface of the dermis.

Step 8

To tighten the skin, I then carefully resurface the undersurface of the dermis in a crisscrossing randomized fashion, using the UltraPulse 5000 laser on a 7-W defocused setting (Fig. 9-6). Care must be taken to keep the laser beam moving continuously. The amount of resurfacing done on the undersurface of the skin will depend on the skin laxity, the skin thickness, and the amount of tightening desired. Resurfacing should only be done on 20% to 30% of the skin undersurface, rather than a total or dense pattern as is used with external skin resurfacing procedures. I evert the skin and hold my nondominant "smart" hand behind the area being resurfaced to carefully monitor for any areas of heat, which would indicate excessive laser concentration in a particular area.

Step 9

In patients with slight to moderate microgenia, the mandible may be augmented to maximize the cervicomental angle. The implant procedure is initiated at this time by using the UltraPulse 5000 laser on the 7-W continuous setting to carefully separate the platysma muscle in a horizontal line proceeding down to the periosteum on the mandible, corresponding to the desired position for the implant. The periosteum is then incised with the UltraPulse 5000 laser. A Rich periosteal elevator is utilized to create a pocket subperiosteally along the border of the mandible. The pocket for the implant should be located so that the implant will seat comfortably and squarely over the chin prominence and will not extend higher than the natural labiomental groove. The pocket must accommodate the prosthesis comfortably; otherwise, the implant will slide inferiorly over the symphysis and rock back and forth.

Once the pocket is freed and hemostasis is achieved, the implant is positioned and is secured to the periosteum with 4-0 clear nylon sutures. The fibers of the platysma muscle are then reapproximated with 4-0 Vicryl sutures. This fixes the implant in place and helps to prevent malposition and extrusion.

Step 10

Platysmal tightening is then performed to additionally improve the cervicomental angle and to reduce neck banding. After liposuction, severing of the septae, and removal of the platysmal insertions into the skin of the neck, the pattern of the particular individual's platysma muscle can clearly be noted. Because of the support given by the platysma and its role in the creation of the cervicomental angle, there is no substitute for a thorough plication of the medial platysma to create the best results in the neck.

The medial borders of the platysma muscle are carefully sutured together using a plication stitch of 3-0 Vicryl. I prefer a vertical mattress type of suture, which gives better strength to the plicated muscle so that it will heal firmly. By the time the suture is absorbed, there will be a good firm support of the muscular filaments and the overlying fascia. Nonabsorbable suture material in this area is not as effective, because it may cause irritation, infection, or extrusion of the sutures.

The number of sutures and their placement will vary considerably, depending on the anatomy of the underlying platysma muscle. In some individuals the muscle is quite thick, and when the suture is placed, a ridge may develop in the midline. Using the UltraPulse 5000 laser to smooth out any surface irregularities can easily decrease the fullness of this ridge. One must be cautious to lase only the elevated portion of the muscle and not to lase over the sutures that have been already positioned.

Below the point of plication, a small wedge of muscle is resected from each of the anterior platysmal borders to break the continuity of the band and allow the creation of a sharp cervicomental angle. This allows the muscle to conform to the cervicomental angle rather than forming a "bowstring" across it.

With good hemostasis achieved in all areas, the submental incision is closed with 4-0 Vicryl in the subcutaneous layer and 5-0 running and interrupted clear Prolene sutures in the skin surface (Fig. 9-7). As with all my liposculpture procedures, the remaining scissors stab incisions in the infra-auricular and lip areas are left open to promote drainage.

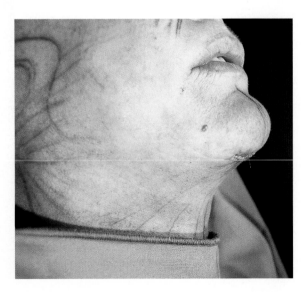

Figure 9-7

Immediate postoperative result of the Cook Weekend Alternative to the Facelift™.

▷ Postoperative Considerations

Stretch foam tape (3M, St. Paul, Minn.) is applied to the neck and lower facial areas. The stretch foam tape must be positioned very carefully so as not to induce any folds in the skin. An initial row of tape is positioned in the midline of the neck. Strips of approximately 8 to 10 cm in length are carefully laid down on the anterior aspect of the neck. Then strips of tape are attached to the midline tape and extended up laterally at approximately 45 degrees over the mandible to the lower one-third of the face. Again, one must be extremely careful not to fold the skin at the lateral aspect of the incisional line. If the stretch foam tape is overtightened so as to produce a fold in the skin, the fold may become semipermanent or permanent. The tape is then covered by elastic neck support with Velcro attachments to hold the tissues in the appropriate position (Fig. 9-8).

On returning home, the patient is advised to rest for the remainder of the day, with the head elevated and ice packs in position over the lower face and neck, 15 minutes "on" and 15 minutes "off." This will help to reduce tissue swelling and prevent ecchymosis of the areas. Good hydration should be maintained through adequate water intake. (See Table 4-8 for postoperative instructions following this procedure.)

The first full postoperative day should be spent in quiet activities, with periodic rest, head elevation, and application of ice packs. Patients are instructed to leave the tape in place until the surgeon or his or her assistant removes it in 1 to 2 days, and to wear the chinstrap 8 to 12 hours a day for 1 week. Excessive activity too soon after surgery is not recommended.

After 1 to 2 days patients return to the office for removal of the tape (Figs. 9-9 to 9-11). Patients are advised to shower just before coming to the office; this will loosen the tape and facilitate its removal.

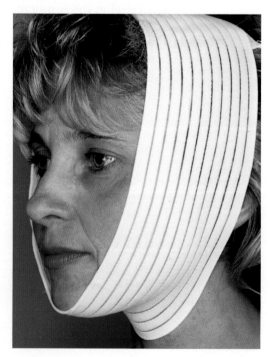

Figure 9-8

Chin strap worn following the Cook Weekend Alternative to the Facelift™.

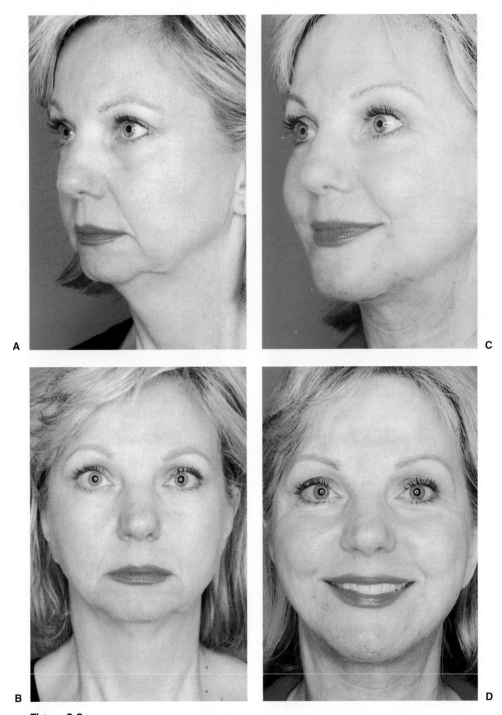

Figure 9-9

Patient (**A,B**) before surgery and (**C,D**) 2 days after the Cook Weekend Alternative to the Facelift™ with chin implant. Note redness immediately following tape removal.

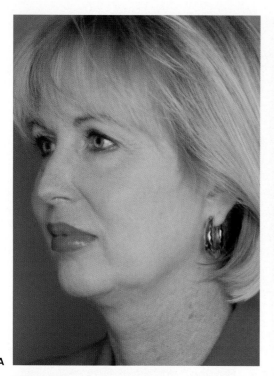
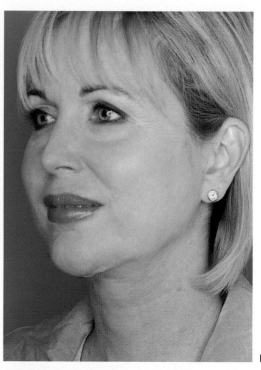

A   B

Figure 9-10

Patient (**A**) before and (**B**) 3 days after the Cook Weekend Alternative to the Facelift™ with chin implant. Note submental sutures with sterile strips (Steri-strips) still in place.

After this, patients can return to work and normal activities (Fig. 9-11). However, vigorous exercise or physical exertion should be avoided for approximately 1 week following surgery. Immersion in water such as a swimming pool, hot tub, or bath must be avoided until all the incisions have closed and the sutures are removed.

The sutures should be left in place for 14 to 21 days, to assure good healing of the area and good approximation of the wound. We have found that this extended period of suture retention is needed because of the tissue contracture that occurs following the dermal resurfacing with the UltraPulse 5000 laser. This contracture, along with movement of the area, places a great deal of stress on the healing wound. If a chin implant has been inserted, this will increase the stress on the wound because of normal postoperative swelling. Premature removal of the sutures may result in wound dehiscence. Because I use clear 5-0 Prolene suture, the sutures cause only minimal cosmetic inconvenience to the patient.

Patients undergoing this procedure generally experience no to minimal postoperative ecchymosis and usually no postoperative discomfort. Occasionally, the chin implant site may be tender for 1 to 2 days postoperatively. Patients are usually able to return to work and social activities on the third postoperative day. Exercise of any strenuous type should be avoided for the first week postoperatively.

Although the procedure allows the patient to have significant surgical intervention with very rapid recovery, the final result of the surgical procedure will not be apparent for 2 to 3 months postoperatively. This must be emphasized before

(text continues on page 87)

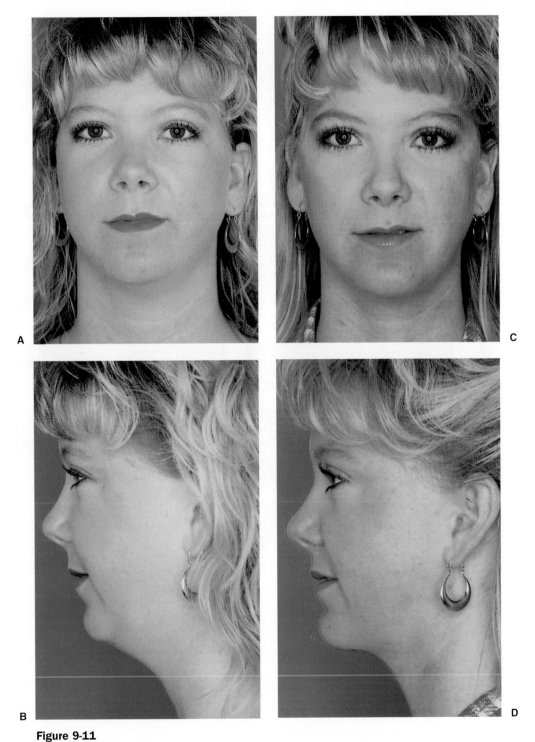

Figure 9-11
Patient (**A,B**) before surgery and (**C,D**) 3 days after the Cook Weekend Alternative to the Facelift™ with chin implant, immediately following tape removal.

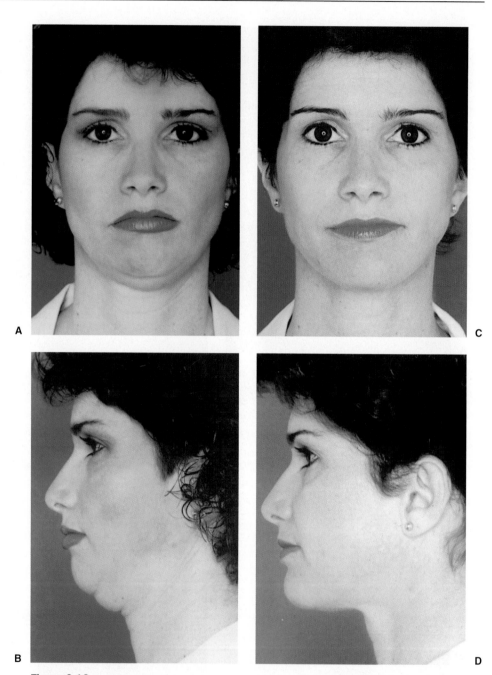

Figure 9-12
Patient (**A,B**) before surgery and (**C,D**) after the Cook Weekend Alternative to the
Facelift™ with chin implant.

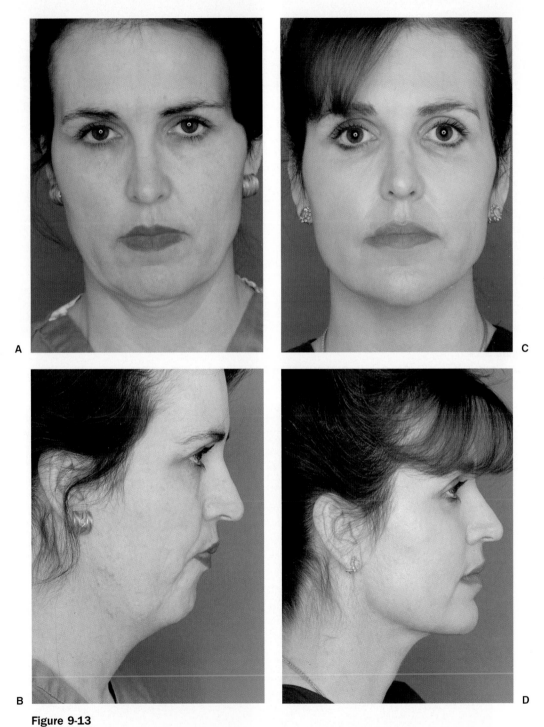

Figure 9-13

Patient (**A,B**) before surgery and (**C,D**) after the Cook Weekend Alternative to the Facelift™ with chin implant.

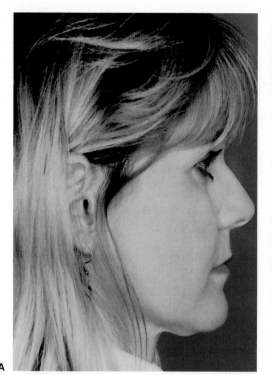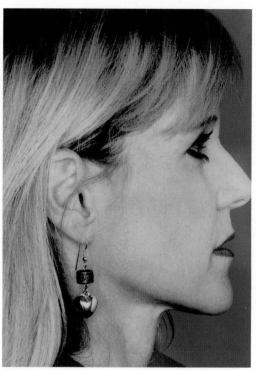

A
B

Figure 9-14

Patient (**A**) before and (**B**) after the Cook Weekend Alternative to the Facelift™ without chin implant.

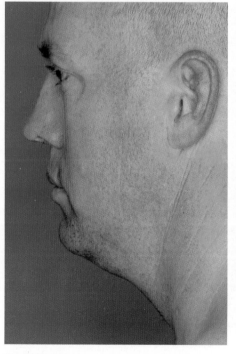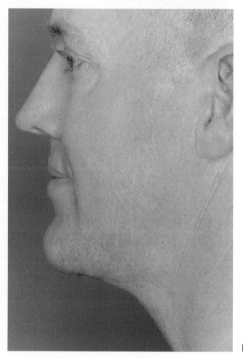

A
B

Figure 9-15

Patient (**A**) before and (**B**) 3 days after the Cook Weekend Alternative to the Facelift™ with chin implant.

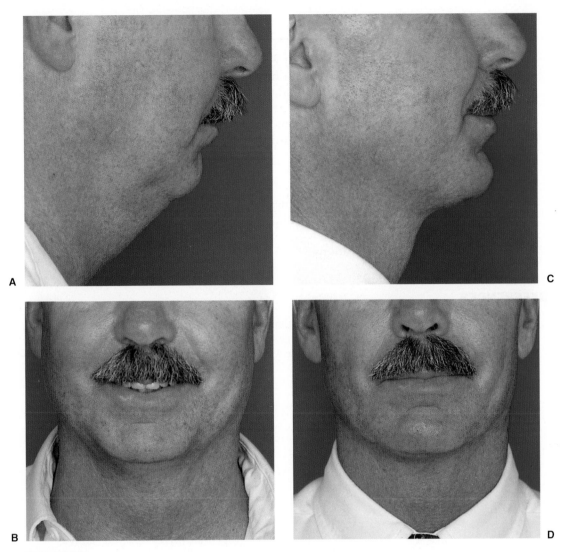

Figure 9-16
Patient (**A,B**) before and (**C,D**) after the Cook Weekend Alternative to the Facelift™ with chin implant.

the operation, so that the patient's expectations will be in line with the natural healing processes that will take place.

We have had no permanent complications to date. Some individuals will recover more rapidly than others, depending on the amount of skin retraction that must occur. Rarely, a small seroma may develop during the postoperative period. These may easily be drained, and recovery will then proceed uneventfully with excellent clinical results.

Individuals with a history of keloid formation need to be monitored and treated with intralesional triamcinolone (Kenalog) as indicated. (See Table 4-2 for a more complete listing of possible sequelae and complications.)

▷ Results

After this procedure (Figs. 9-12 to 9-16), patients with round and heavy appearing faces gain a slimmer look with more prominent appearing cheekbones. The cervicomental angle is excellent and the mandible is more sharply defined. Overall, the facial features are in better balance.

In summary, the Cook Weekend Alternative to the Facelift™ offers the following advantages over liposculpture alone or traditional rhytidectomy:

- ▶ Rapid recovery
- ▶ Excellent cosmetic results
- ▶ Done entirely under local anesthesia
- ▶ Little to no postoperative discomfort
- ▶ Minimal incisions
- ▶ Minimal complications

REFERENCES

1. Farkas LG, Sohm P, Kolar JC, Katic MJ, Munro IR. Inclinations of the facial profile: art versus reality. *Plast Reconstr Surg* 1985;75:509–519
2. Farkas LG, Kolar JC. Anthropometrics and art in the aesthetics of women's faces. *Clin Plast Surg* 1987;14:599–616.

CHAPTER 10

LIPOSCULPTURE OF THE ABDOMEN, FLANKS, WAIST, AND INFRASCAPULAR AREA: THREE-DIMENSIONAL TUMESCENT LIPOSCULPTURE™

Preoperative Evaluation ▶ *Surgical Procedure* ▶ *Postoperative Considerations* ▶ *Results*

Liposculpture of the abdomen, flanks, and waist is a very fulfilling procedure for the patient and the surgeon. When performed as described on appropriately selected patients, it yields consistently good results and a high level of patient satisfaction.

In sculpting the torso, it is important to regard the entire area as a cosmetic unit and to treat it with what I call "Three-Dimensional Tumescent Liposculpture™." Simply removing isolated pockets of fat from the abdomen, hips, or waist will not achieve a pleasing cosmetic result, and in fact may leave the patient with a bodily appearance that is seriously out of balance. Proper tumescent liposculpture of the torso shapes the body, rather than merely removing the fat. The surgeon must consider the abdomen, flanks, waist, and, if present, the infrascapular fat pad as a three-dimensional unit and plan the surgical procedure accordingly. If this is done skillfully, patients' bodies will be in better proportion, clothing will fit better, and patients will achieve a firmer and more youthful contour consistent with their body type, age, and level of fitness.

The abdomen, flanks, waist, and infrascapular areas, if needed, can be conveniently treated in a single surgical procedure under tumescent local anesthesia. If treatment of the buttocks and/or thighs is also needed, a separate procedure should be planned. The two procedures should be carefully designed to complement each other, so that the ultimate cosmetic result will be a well-balanced body with all areas in proportion to each other. See Chapters 11, 12, and 13 for several different surgical approaches to the buttocks and upper legs. See Chapter 15 for a discussion of the arms and axillary folds, which may be sculpted as a unit with the back. See Chapter 16 for a discussion of liposculpture of the male chest.

Women typically refer to the flank areas as their hips, and men call them the "love handles," but the area is important to males and females. Males very seldom need to have the lateral thigh area treated, but some men have excessive lipodystrophic changes in the buttocks, which can be helped by liposculpture. For the most part, however, male patients will usually be treated as described in this chapter, while females more commonly need a procedure that focuses on the flanks, lateral thighs, and buttocks (see Chapter 11).

The surgeon must consider the factors that will influence the number of areas to treat. In all cases, the total milligrams of lidocaine infused should be kept within safe limits.

▷ Preoperative Evaluation

Ideal candidates for this procedure are within 10 to 20 pounds of their ideal body weight and in good health. Ideally they should have good skin elasticity, eat a balanced diet, and be on a regular exercise program.

Patients who do not fit these ideal criteria can still benefit from liposculpture, provided the limitations are clearly explained. All ages may be considered for the procedure. Patients who are 20 to 30 pounds over their ideal body weight but otherwise meet the criteria can achieve good results from liposculpture. Patients must realize that this procedure is not a "quick fix" and does not substitute for a proper regimen of diet and exercise.

Some practitioners are using mega-liposuction as a treatment for obesity. However, this chapter will address only the use of liposculpture on patients who fit these previously described criteria.

For patients who are more than 30 pounds over their ideal body weight, I sometimes perform the Cook Weekend Alternative to the Facelift™ on the face, neck, and jowls (see Chapter 9) and/or liposculpture of the arms (see Chapter 15). The resulting improvement in appearance often motivates them to lose weight through diet and exercise, so that they become better candidates for body liposculpture. As with any liposculpture, patients who have recently lost a great deal of weight (100 pounds or more) may not receive a great deal of benefit from this procedure because of poor elasticity of the skin.

Patients need to understand the limitations of the surgery. It is important to maintain good muscle tone after surgery. Bony structure will remain the same. Previous scars will not be eliminated, although the puckering around them may be greatly improved and the depression elevated. Striae distensae will persist; however, they may become less noticeable because they are not stretched out by the excess fat. Skin elasticity will not change. Liposculpture is not a treatment for so-called "cellulite," although superficial breaking of the connective tissue fibers may result in a decrease in this condition (see Chapter 13).

Physical examination should be performed with the patient unclothed in a standing position. Evaluate and note the patient's overall weight, muscle development, skin tone, and any scars, ventral or other hernias, or asymmetry. Perform a pinch test to determine if the problem is in the subcutaneous fatty tissue or in the intraabdominal fat pad. Fat that is intraabdominal rather than subcutaneous, a condition that is more common in males, is not treatable by liposculpture. A subcutaneous thickness of 3 cm or more usually indicates that the patient can benefit from the procedure; however, each patient should be evaluated on an individual basis.

Patients who have very poor skin elasticity may need to be referred for abdominoplasty.

▷ Surgical Procedure

The operative area should be carefully marked with a gentian violet marking pen with the patient in a standing position (Figs. 10-1, 10-2). The surgeon should be aware of an important area of depression that may be present inferior to the lateral flanks, called the lateral gluteal depression (Fig. 10-1; see also Fig. 11-1). This depression is caused by fascial connections from the superficial fascial system to the deep muscle fascia. This depression delineates the inferior border of the lateral flank. Other landmarks, which should be identified, include the inframammary crease; the vertical midline from the midbreasts to the pubis; and the horizontal midline through the umbilicus.

The markings should indicate the location and extent of particular areas of lipodystrophy. In women, these areas may include a roll of fat below the breasts; a double-bulge contour of the lateral flank (Fig. 10-2B), with particular attention given to the location of the natural lateral gluteal depression just below it; the strip of adiposity running from the lateral flank to the midback waistline (Fig. 10-2C); the infrascapular fat pad running from the inframammary crease to the midback (Fig. 10-2C); and the presacral fat pad. In men, the same areas need to be addressed, but the love handles are usually located more superiorly, above the iliac crest. Also, men usually do not have infrascapular fat pads.

Incision sites should also be marked at this time. For suctioning the abdomen I prefer to use three incisions in the suprapubic area, one in the midline and two laterally, as well as one incision at the superior margin of the umbilicus. These incisions will provide good postoperative drainage and allow for adequate crisscrossing of the lower abdomen. Two or three incisions are placed on each side of the abdomen along the anterior axillary line: a superior lateral abdominal incision, an anterior waistline incision, and a lower lateral

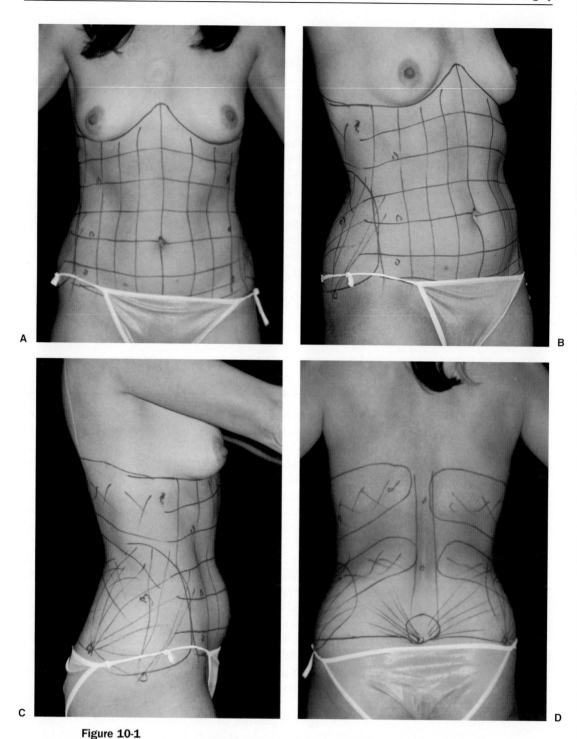

Figure 10-1

A-D: Patient marked for liposculpture surgery of the abdomen, flanks, waist, infrascapular area, and sacral fat pad, showing incision sites. In **A**, note the lateral gluteal depression just below the right lateral flank.

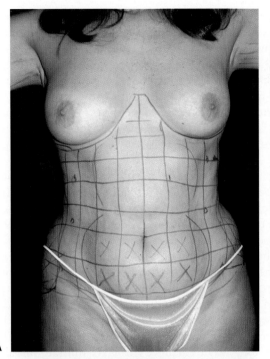
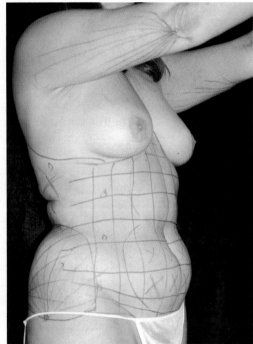
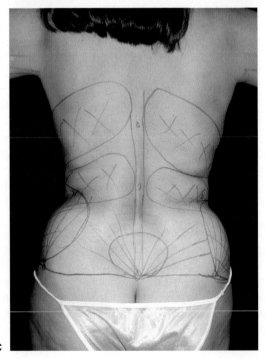

Figure 10-2

A-C: Patient marked for liposculpture surgery of the abdomen, flanks, waist, infrascapular area, sacral fat pad, and arms. Note "X" marks for increased areas of adiposity.

abdominal incision. For treatment of the lateral flanks I use five incision sites: two inferior flank incisions just superior to the lateral gluteal depression, the previously mentioned anterior waistline incision, the previously mentioned lower lateral abdominal incision, and a lateral waistline incision. For treatment of the sacral area, posterior flanks, and infrascapular area, I additionally use a superior posterior axillary line incision, a midline infrascapular incision, a midline posterior flank incision, and a midline presacral incision. The incisions are staggered slightly to make them less obvious during the postoperative healing phase. Because the incision sites are so small, they virtually disappear in the majority of patients.

After marking, the patient is placed in the supine position and infiltrated with tumescent solution. I generally use solution with a 0.1% lidocaine concentration for the abdomen and 0.05% lidocaine for the flanks and infrascapular area. See Chapter 5 for formulation of the tumescent solution and general considerations regarding the use of tumescent local anesthesia. The most important consideration in the use of tumescent anesthesia is the total dosage of lidocaine delivered to the individual. I aim for an upper limit of 60 mg/kg of body weight. The initial infiltration should deliver less than this amount, in the range of 40 to 50 mg/kg, to allow for additional infiltration during the case if necessary to provide additional anesthesia or to expand the space and achieve better sculpting capability. In a smaller individual, I attempt to reduce the estimated maximum amount of lidocaine to approximately 50 mg/kg. One way to achieve this is to infiltrate initially with tumescent solution of 0.05% concentration and then, just before beginning the sculpting, to reinfiltrate with a small amount of 0.1% solution for final anesthesia of the areas. Small amounts (up to 2 mL) to 1% to 2% lidocaine with epinephrine 1:100,000 are injected around the umbilicus to reduce tenderness in this sensitive area.

When anesthesia is complete, external ultrasound can be given if indicated (see Chapter 6). Suctioning of the abdomen is begun approximately 20 minutes or more after infiltration, to allow time for vasoconstriction to occur.

I start with a 14-gauge Klein spatula cannula, with the two ports always placed in a downward position. As surgery progresses, I increase to a 12-gauge Klein spatula cannula, a 3-mm Pinto cannula, a 3-mm Cook cannula, and finally I complete sculpting of the area with a smaller 12-gauge Klein spatula cannula. The larger 3.5-mm and occasionally 4-mm cannulas are primarily used in large volume body reduction cases.

Suctioning of one side of the abdomen is begun from the three lateral abdominal incision sites in a fairly deep plane. Use of the deep plane permits the surgeon to determine the firmness of the various areas of the adipose layer, establish early tunneling, and develop a pattern for removal of fat. These lateral incisions are helpful to establish good crisscrossing and to remove fat from the upper and lower abdomen. Beginning on the lateral aspect provides good access and helps to establish an adequate tissue plane.

One must suction carefully deep to Scarpa's fascia. I begin with a 4-inch 14-gauge Klein cannula, then a 6-inch 14-gauge Capistrano cannula. If the adipose layer is extremely firm or cicatricial, this initial suctioning will significantly soften the area. It is then possible to switch to a 3-mm Pinto cannula for more definitive suctioning of fibrous areas, or a 3-mm Cook cannula for less fibrous areas and for feathering into adjacent areas. When the first side of the abdomen is adequately treated at the deep level, I repeat the procedure on the contralateral side.

If any depressed scars are present, I elevate them by using a Toledo tissue dissector superficially just below the skin. The elevation should be done carefully, and the surgeon may want to observe the thickness of the scar. This will permit the scar tissue to rise to the same level as the surrounding areas that were just sculpted. If it appears that the scar may not be easily released from underlying structures, I do not attempt to elevate it.

Next, I utilize the supraumbilical incision site to suction the upper and lower abdomen, emphasizing the periumbilical fat pad. I begin with a 4-inch Klein spatula cannula, either 12 or 14 gauge, followed by a 6-inch Klein spatula cannula. Through this supraumbilical incision, I use a clockwise pattern around the umbilicus to adequately remove the periumbilical "fat donut," which should be carefully suctioned.

I then return to the lower abdominal incisions and perform midplane and relatively superficial liposculpture with a 12-gauge Klein cannula. This removes the remainder of the lower abdominal fat pad to create as smooth an abdomen as possible.

I always feather into the suprapubic area. However, in cases where the suprapubic fat pad is thick, it may need additional attention. The area should be suctioned comparably to the degree of suctioning given the abdomen; otherwise the suprapubic area may appear excessively large postoperatively. I use two additional incisions, which are lateral pubic incisions located superior to the inguinal crease, 2 to 3 cm medial to the femoral pulse. I use a 4-inch 14-gauge Klein cannula followed by a 4-inch 12-gauge Klein cannula to crisscross the area.

The patient is then turned on the side to permit treatment of the lateral flank and waist. Using the two inferior flank incisions and the lower lateral abdominal incision, the area is sculpted in a crisscrossing pattern. Then the waist is sculpted from the anterior waistline and lateral waistline incisions, carefully dissecting deep and superficial components. When sculpting the waist, it is important that the suctioning be deep to Scarpa's fascia in that area, so that an attractive waistline can be produced. The object is to form a uniformly sloping curve of a natural waistline. Suctioning is continued in the posterior flank, first from the anterior waistline incision, then from the lateral waistline incision. This fat pad, which runs at approximately a 45-degree angle upward under the back, must be removed thoroughly. By suctioning deep to Scarpa's fascia and sculpting the posterior flank, the surgeon can produce a dramatically reduced waistline, which is preferred by many patients and has been called the "Cook waist."

Next, the lateral portion of the infrascapular fat pad is treated from the superior lateral abdominal incision. Then the patient is tilted slightly toward the surgeon and the medial portion of the infrascapular fat pad is treated from the superior posterior axillary line incision.

The patient is then turned to the contralateral side and the procedure is repeated.

Finally, the patient is placed in the prone position. Final reduction of the infrascapular fat pad and posterior flank is achieved through the midline infrascapular incision and the posterior flank incision.

Next, the presacral fat pad is suctioned. The presacral fat pad can produce significant anatomic deformity in many patients. A thick and large presacral fat pad may add several inches to the patient's circumferential measurements and is very important in the overall fit of clothing. Therefore, it should be thoroughly suctioned at this point using the following method: A small stab incision is made midline in the inferior aspect of the presacral fat pad just above the gluteal crease. Through this midline presacral fat pad incision, suctioning is begun, generally with a 4-inch 14-gauge Klein cannula. This helps to break up this very fibrofatty fat pad. Following this, the 3-mm Pinto cannula is very efficient in removing the remainder of the fat pad. Through this incision and one of the inferior flank incisions, suctioning can also be done to feather the junction line between the posterior flank and the superior aspect of the buttocks. Usually a 12-gauge Klein spatula cannula is effective for this feathering.

▷ Postoperative Considerations

When the procedure is completed and good hemostasis is achieved, all areas are cleansed and an antibiotic ointment may be applied. An absorbent dressing and then a compression surgical garment are put on (Figs. 10-3, 10-4).

The garment should be of a type to produce good firm compression for the immediate postoperative period. This compression will help to reduce swelling, expel the excess tumescent solution, promote hemostasis, and also provide comfort for the patient. Overcompression is not necessary. The initially firm degree of compression will naturally decrease over the next 24 to 48 hours as tumescent solution is expelled and swelling is reduced.

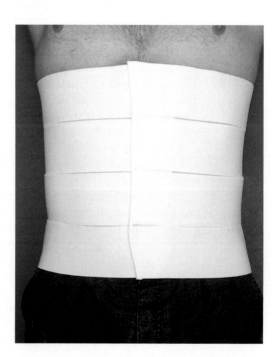

Figure 10-3

Male patient wearing a binder after liposculpture of the abdomen, flanks, and waist.

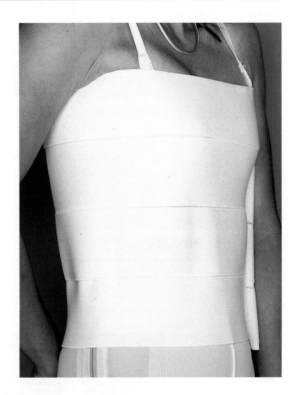

Figure 10-4

Female patient wearing a binder and above-the-knee garment after liposculpture of the abdomen, flanks, waist, and infrascapular area.

For the rest of the day following surgery, patients are advised to rest, drink plenty of fluids to maintain good hydration, and eat light meals. The garment is left in place for approximately 12 hours postoperatively. If the absorbent dressings become moist from drainage, they can be slipped out from under the garment and appropriate dry pads can be positioned in their place. Patients generally wear the surgical garment 12 to 23 hours per day for the first week. During weeks 2 and 3, they wear the garment electively as they see fit. Because of the comfort the garment provides, most patients elect to wear the garment for 2 to 3 weeks postoperatively, but they may wear it for a shorter period of time.

On the first postoperative day, the patient's first priority is generally a shower. Patients should have someone assist them when they remove the garment, in case they become slightly light-headed. They should be well hydrated prior to removal of the garment. Patients will shower with chlorhexidine gluconate (Hibiclens) solution, then cover the incision sites with clean absorbent dressings and put on a clean, dry surgical garment. It must be stressed that patients avoid water immersion in a bathtub, Jacuzzi, or swimming pool. They may take as many showers as they like.

Next, I recommend that patients take a 2-mile walk. I find this early walk to be extremely important in the recovery process. This type of movement helps to expel excess tumescent solution, reduce tissue edema, and expedite the patient's recovery. Patients should consume a normal diet, low in salt so as not to promote any tissue edema. Of course, they should take their antibiotics and other medications as prescribed.

The average patient on the second full postoperative day will resume normal activities, returning to work if desired and continuing with light exercise, such as walking. Strenuous activity following liposculpture should be resumed gradually, depending on the patient's age, previous conditioning, level of exercise done preoperatively, and other factors, which the surgeon and the patient should discuss. Generally, at the end of the first week most patients are able to perform any strenuous activities that they had performed on a regular basis preoperatively.

▷ Results

Postoperatively (Figs. 10-5 to 10-12), patients display a flatter abdomen, a better defined waist, reduction of love handles, and reduction of the infrascapular bulge.

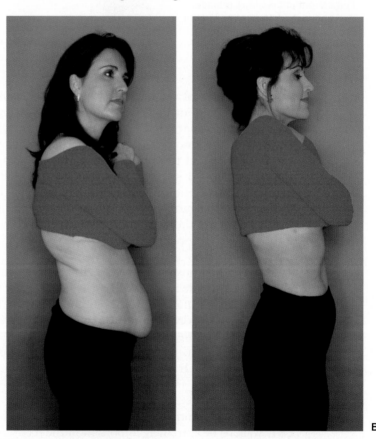

A   B

Figure 10-5

Female patient (**A**) before and (**B**) 3 weeks after liposculpture of the abdomen, flanks, waist, and infrascapular area.

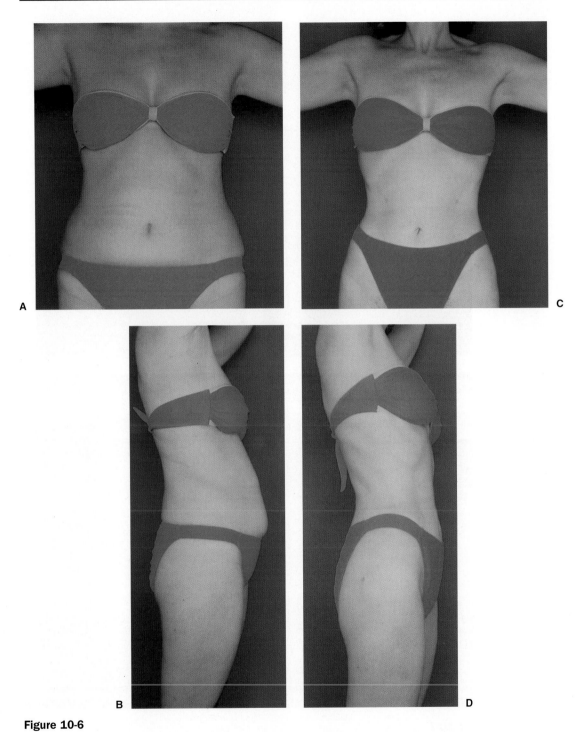

Figure 10-6

Female patient (**A,B**) before and (**C,D**) after liposculpture of the abdomen, flanks, waist, and infrascapular area.

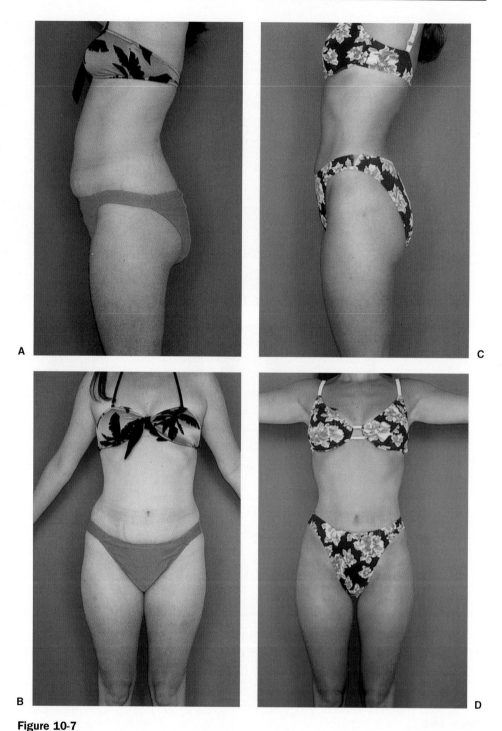

Figure 10-7

Female patient (**A,B**) before and (**C,D**) after liposculpture of the abdomen, flanks, waist, and infrascapular area.

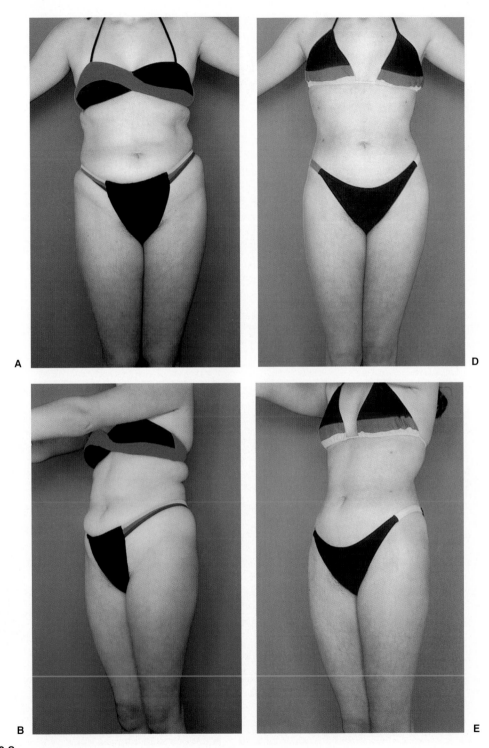

Figure 10-8

Female patient (**A–C**) before and (**D–F**) after liposculpture of the abdomen, flanks, waist, and infrascapular area. *(continued)*

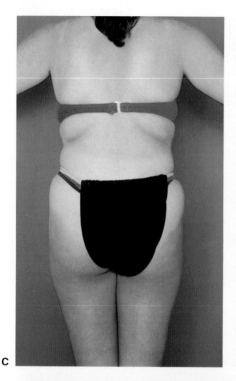

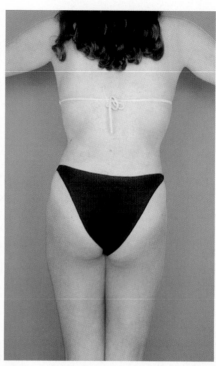

C

F

Figure 10-8
(continued)

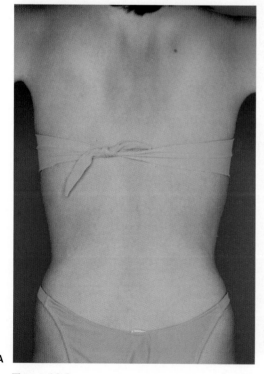

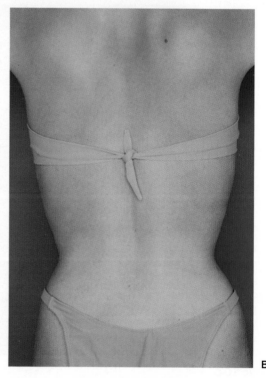

A

B

Figure 10-9

Female patient (**A**) before and (**B**) after liposculpture of the abdomen, flanks, waist, and infrascapular area. Note that fat was suctioned beneath Scarpa's fascia to produce a small waistline.

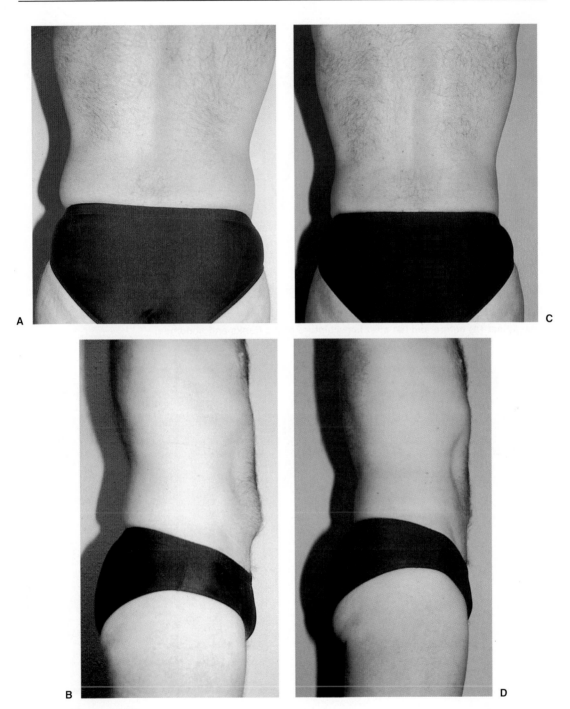

Figure 10-10
Male patient (**A,B**) before and (**C,D**) after liposculpture of the flanks and abdomen.

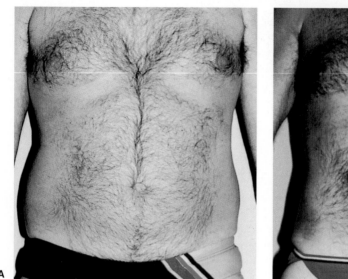
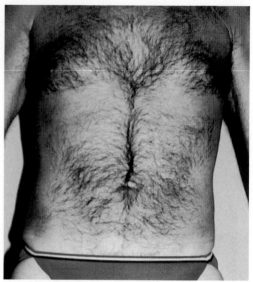

A B

Figure 10-11
Male patient (**A**) before and (**B**) after liposculpture of the flanks and abdomen.

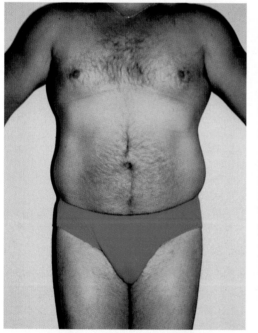
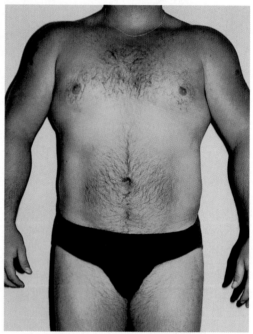

A B

Figure 10-12
Male patient (**A**) before and (**B**) after liposculpture of the flanks and abdomen.

CHAPTER 11

LIPOSCULPTURE OF THE FLANKS, THIGHS, AND BUTTOCKS: THREE-DIMENSIONAL TUMESCENT LIPOSCULPTURE™

Preoperative Evaluation ▶ *Surgical Procedure* ▶
Postoperative Considerations ▶ *Results*

The flank areas should be treated as part of a three-dimensional cosmetic unit, either with the abdomen or with the buttocks and lateral thighs, depending on the pattern of lipodystrophy in the patient. In both cases, the flanks should be included in the sculpting to achieve the optimal cosmetic appearance, appropriate fit of clothing, and maximal long-term results.

One of the most common technical errors is to randomly suction one or more of these areas without considering their interrelationship. For example, the effect of gravity pulls downward through this plane from the flank and contributes to ptosis of the buttocks. The weight of the buttocks, in turn, often produces significant bulging of the lateral thigh area. The effect that one area has on another should be discussed in the preoperative consultation.

The surgeon should first consider the flanks in their relationship with the adjacent abdomen, lateral thighs, and buttocks. This chapter is devoted to individuals who have lipodystrophy primarily of the lower half of the body—the flanks, buttocks, and thighs. For individuals who have lipodystrophy primarily in the abdomen, the flanks should be considered an integral part of that cosmetic unit and treated as described in Chapter 10.

Women typically refer to the flank areas as their hips, and men call them the "love handles." But, basically, there is substantial overlap anatomically, and the importance for men and women cannot be overlooked. Men seldom need the lateral thigh area treated. However, some men have excessive lipodystrophic changes in the buttocks, which can be helped by liposculpture. For convenience, the male flank areas are discussed in Chapter 10. In this chapter, we will primarily focus on the woman who needs sculpting of the flanks, lateral thighs, and buttocks.

The lateral and posterior flanks, lateral thighs, and the buttocks should be considered an anatomic unit in most individuals with lipodystrophy of the lower half of the body. Patients often present with complaints other than the flank areas, not realizing their importance and interrelationship with adjacent regions. It is the surgeon's responsibility to point out this interrelationship so that the patient can obtain optimal cosmetic results. By contouring all of these contiguous areas in a three-dimensional manner, the patient will be given not only immediate cosmetic relief, but also a more lasting cosmetic result due to the overall reduction of the adipose layers. Because these regions traditionally tend to increase in size as a unit if the patient should gain weight in the future, treating the entire area as an anatomic unit should give the patient a much better long-term cosmetic result.

▷ Preoperative Evaluation

Female patients will often present with a complaint of protrusion of the lateral thighs, the so-called "saddlebag" region. The surgeon should also evaluate the lateral and posterior flanks and buttocks to determine their interrelation and the contribution of each section to the overall region. Considering them as a cosmetic unit will permit the surgeon to sculpt this region uniformly and leave the patient with an excellent cosmetic result.

The desired effect is to develop a nice flowing line from the waist down over the iliac crest to the inferior aspect of the lateral thighs. Regional and ethnic considerations must be considered in the preoperative discussion, as well as patient goals and expectations. General surgical principles, current fashion trends, and the ideal body configuration that is continually displayed by the media will give the surgeon guidelines for discussion and help to elicit the patient's expectations.

There is an important lateral gluteal depression that may be present above the lateral thigh and sometimes in the lateral buttocks in women (Fig. 11-1). In men, this depression is usually more superior in position, located at the iliac crest just below the so-called love handles. This depression is caused by fascial connections from the superficial fascial system to the deep muscle fascia. This landmark varies in intensity from individual to individual. It can be evaluated and discussed with patients during the initial consultation. By having patients contract the buttocks maximally during examination, the surgeon can more clearly see the outline of this region and, therefore, determine the area where only minimal or light liposculpture should be performed. The incisions are made at the four corners of this de-

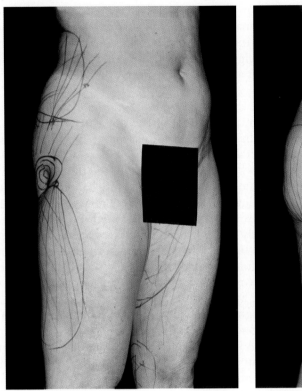 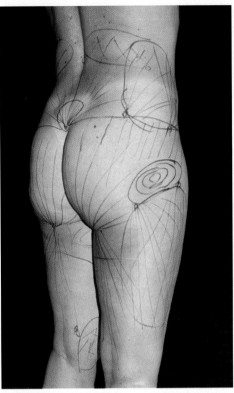

A   B

Figure 11-1
Preoperative markings for liposculpture, showing the lateral gluteal depression indicated by
the concentric circle. **A, B** are two different patients.

pressed site, and suctioning within the depressed area itself is generally avoided.
The physician should mark this depression preoperatively and may want to avoid
aggressive suctioning in this area. As mentioned previously (see Chapter 7), I outline depressions by concentric circles within circles.

The buttocks should be evaluated to determine their relative weight or density, the amount of protrusion of the buttock curve, and the amount of ptosis present. When the patient is told to contract the buttocks tightly, one can readily assess the role of the buttocks in causing the lateral thighs to protrude, because this
protrusion will be significantly diminished when the buttocks are contracted. The
result of a general volume reduction of the buttocks will be to relieve some of the
downward and outward pressure they exert on the lateral thigh area. If the surgeon fails to consider the role of the buttocks in causing the lateral thigh protrusion and treats the lateral thighs alone, the result may be an inferior cosmetic out-
come. Either a depression in the lateral thigh can result, where too much lateral
thigh fat pad was suctioned, or possible persistent bulging may remain, even after
the majority of the lateral thigh fat pad was eliminated, because too little was suctioned from the buttock.

The presacral fat pad can contribute extensively to the overall waist dimension
in some individuals and should not be neglected.

The upper posterior thighs in many individuals have a predominant fatty fold, which has been coined the "banana roll." It is important to address this region during the preoperative consultation and in the surgical procedure. Smoothing this region will help relieve this bulge and additionally accentuate the normal aesthetic curve of the buttocks, with a flattening or more desirable contour of the posterior thigh region in general.

It is always important to leave the natural rounding of the gluteal region and not to flatten the buttocks. In many patients, the lateral thigh area will overlap and continue onto the posterior thighs. This is an ideal time to treat the posterior thighs as well, to obtain good overall contouring.

The question may arise as to whether to treat more of the thigh than just the lateral and posterior portions. As noted in greater detail in Chapter 13, sculpting the entire circumference of the thigh in a single procedure may produce a higher degree of postoperative swelling. If the patient has large medial thighs, while the rest of the thigh region is relatively normal or only slightly enlarged, the medial thighs may be treated at the same time as the flanks, lateral thighs, and buttocks. However, it is necessary to carefully evaluate the patient's weight, the overall amount of fatty tissue that it is necessary to remove, and the amount of lidocaine that would be required to provide anesthesia for this area.

If the patient has very large thighs overall, the surgeon should plan a two-stage procedure. On the first occasion, one may treat the flanks, buttocks, lateral thighs, and posterior thighs, if necessary. A second, separate procedure may be performed later to treat the medial thighs, anterior thighs, and knees. The second procedure is typically done 2 or more weeks after the first procedure. (See Chapter 13 for a description of the latter procedure.)

Some patients have a very large muscle mass in the lower extremities, combined with a small upper body and small waist. These patients must be counseled that there are limitations to what can be achieved by sculpting, which removes only the fatty deposits. Postoperatively, these patients should plan to pursue a good, modest exercise program, including bicycle or stair-stepping exercises, to produce maximal tightening of the overlying skin and keep the muscles toned and conditioned. But patients with a large muscle mass should be advised not to persist in doing heavy weight lifting and squatting exercises, which can increase the muscle mass and additionally distort the size discrepancy between the upper and lower body. Instead, they should favor high-repetition, low-weight exercises, which tend to make the muscles stronger, tighten the axis between the fascia and the skin, and keep the muscles as lean as possible.

It is important to note preoperatively any asymmetries that may exist between the left and right sides of the patient's body. The most typical cause of asymmetry in the flank area is scoliosis of the spine. With careful sculpting of the areas, one can achieve some improvement in this asymmetry, but it may not be possible to achieve complete symmetrical balance. Also, certain congenital anatomic considerations in the thigh areas may cause an asymmetry, which can be partially corrected. Conditions such as polio may leave one side of the body with muscle atrophy and usually some lessening of the adipose component. Increased exercising of one side of the body or trauma to one side may cause asymmetry. More aggressive suctioning of the contralateral side can improve this asymmetry, but again it may be impossible to correct totally.

If there has been trauma to the lateral thigh area, which is not uncommon in athletes or after a severe fall, the adipose region may be extremely fibrous and cicatricial. Such cases will require much more vigorous sculpting in order to achieve the desired result.

▷ Surgical Procedure

Infiltration of the tumescent solution must be done according to a preoperative plan based on the total amount of lidocaine that will be infused during the case. My current goal is to infiltrate the amount of tumescent solution that provides a dose of lidocaine up to approximately 60 mg per kg of body weight (see Chapter 5). However, the upper limit of lidocaine safety has not been determined, and many surgeons have stated usage of greater than 60 mg/kg.

For this anatomic area, I use a combination of 0.05% and 0.1% lidocaine solutions. One must calculate the amount and concentration of solution to be infused in each surgical area, with a careful eye on the total amount of lidocaine being used for the entire procedure.

The operative areas should be marked with a gentian violet pen with the patient in a standing position (Figs. 11-2 to 11-4). It is extremely important to be

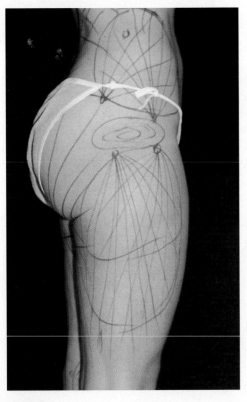
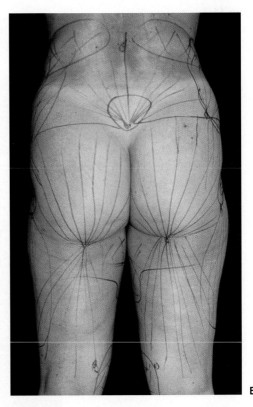

A   B

Figure 11-2

Preoperative markings for liposculpture of the posterior flanks, lateral flanks, presacral areas, buttocks, lateral thighs, posterior thighs, medial thighs, and knees. **A**: side view. **B**: back view.

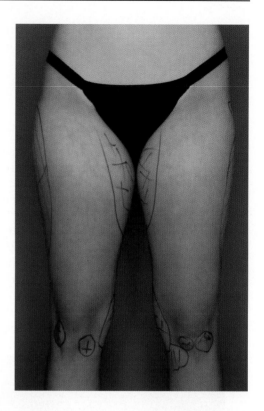

Figure 11-3

Preoperative markings for liposculpture surgery of the medial thighs, lateral thighs, and knees. Front view.

aware of the lateral gluteal depression in planning the surgery (see Fig. 11-1). This region, which lies between the iliac crest and the greater trochanter, contains varying amounts of fatty tissue and generally requires little or no suctioning in order to achieve a single smooth convex curve from the waist to the knee. One must also consider the wedgelike fatty deposit that lies superior and inferior to the lateral infragluteal crease. This deposit can produce a "lateral wedge protrusion," especially when the patient is seated.

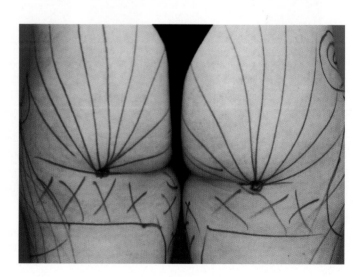

Figure 11-4

Preoperative markings for liposculpture surgery of the "banana roll."

I usually make four incisions surrounding the area of lateral gluteal depression. These allow suctioning upward into the lateral and posterior flank area and downward into the lateral thigh area, achieving good crisscrossing because of the two incision sites in each area. If there is a large amount of subcutaneous tissue in the lateral gluteal depression, light sculpting can be performed in this area to attain the natural desired contour line between the flanks and lateral thigh region.

A lateral waistline incision into the lateral flank area is also very important. Here one can remove the fat that is beneath Scarpa's fascia, obtain maximum definition of the waist, and remove the lateral flank fat pad effectively. Without this lateral waistline incision, complete resolution of the lateral flank may not be nearly as effective.

The posterior flank area runs at a 45-degree angle from approximately the midlateral flanks to the area just lateral to the spine. An incision at the base of the posterior flank in the midline facilitates the removal of the fatty tissue in this region.

The buttocks are accessed through an incision made in the infragluteal crease at the midpoint of each buttock. This same incision is also used to suction the medial thighs. Additional access to the medial thighs is gained through incisions in the lateral pubic area above the inguinal crease. I currently avoid incisions directly in the inguinal crease or in the medial thighs. I have found that scars in these areas may not heal well and may be very visible postoperatively, producing a less desirable cosmetic result than do those in the pubic region.

If the knees are being treated, incisions are made in the area adjacent to the medial knee fat pad posteriorly and also inferiorly. If the patient has fat pads in the infrapatellar region anteriorly, incisions can be made adjacent to those pads laterally and medially. The suprapatellar portion of the anterior knee is not usually sculpted by itself, but rather as part of a treatment of the entire anterior thigh. Performing liposculpture on the suprapatellar area alone may leave a step defect where the treated area adjoins the remaining fat pad in the anterior thigh compartment.

The areas may be treated sequentially as follows:

From the lateral decubitus position: the right lateral flank, right posterior flank, right lateral thigh, left posterior bulge of the medial thigh, and left medial knee.

From the opposite lateral decubitus position: the left lateral flank, left posterior flank, left lateral thigh, right posterior bulge of the medial thigh, and right medial knee.

From the prone position: the buttocks, posterior thighs, and lateral wedge protrusions.

From the supine position: the anterior bulge of the medial thighs and infrapatellar fat pads.

Surgical Procedure for the Lateral and Posterior Flanks

The patient is placed in the lateral decubitus position with the legs together and a pillow between the knees. This tends to take the pressure off the iliotibial band, makes suctioning easier, and facilitates the removal of the deeper fatty components.

I begin treatment of the lateral flank area with a 4-inch 14-gauge Klein spatula cannula. This is a very fibrofatty area, so the initial use of small cannulas facilitates the surgery, acting to break up this fibrofatty area and promoting more effective sculpting of the region. After initial sculpting is achieved with the shorter 14-gauge Klein cannulas, I progress to a 14-gauge Capistrano cannula. Next I use a 3-mm Pinto cannula to suction this fibrofatty area. Complete removal of this area may not be achieved if one uses other cannulas or fails to initially break up the fibrous component with small cannulas. During the suctioning, it is important to attempt to achieve a normal upper body V-shaped contour line, which will extend down to a point overlying the sacrum.

If the presacral fat pad is large, initial suctioning may be done at this time, utilizing a lateral approach from the inferior flank incision. Later, when the patient is in the prone position, I complete the treatment of the presacral area from an incision on the inferior aspect of the presacral fat pad.

The end point for the flank area can be achieved visually and by palpation of the skin-fold thickness. It is important to taper the waistline anteriorly into the adjacent abdominal area so that good blending will occur. This is especially important if the abdomen is not being treated, either at this time or in a subsequent surgery.

Surgical Procedure for the Lateral Thighs

Following the flank liposculpture, attention is given to the lateral thigh area. With the patient still in the lateral decubitus position, the upper leg is bent at a right angle to the trunk, and a pillow is positioned so as to support the leg (Fig. 11-5). This allows the surgeon to approach the lateral thigh of the upper leg from a flat plane and to get a good visual feel for the thickness of the fat pad. In this position,

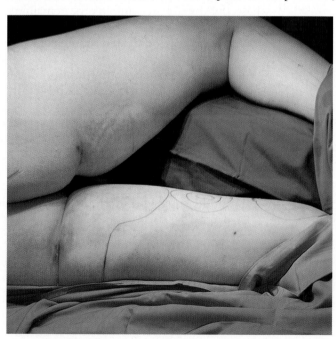

Figure 11-5

Foam surgical pillow positioned to support top leg during liposculpture of the lateral and medial thigh.

uniform suctioning may be achieved from the two lateral thigh incision sites at the inferior poles of the lateral gluteal depression.

Utilizing these two lateral thigh incisions, I begin contouring the whole length of the lateral thigh with 12- or 14-gauge Klein spatula cannulas, gradually increasing from the 4 to 6 inch to 10 to 12 inch lengths, so that pretunneling and initial sculpting can be performed at a midplane or lower depth. It is important not to sculpt too superficially, and especially to stay in the deeper planes at the start of the treatment of this area.

Next, I suction the lateral thigh, using the infragluteal crease incision for blending with the posterior thigh and crisscrossing of the lateral thigh.

Attention is then directed to the upper portion of the lateral thigh through the two lateral thigh incisions. It is not necessary to change the position of the patient. Raising or lowering the table will give the surgeon good access to the area and keep the planes of contouring in clear view and good perspective. One should not subdivide the areas too drastically, since that can lead to oversculpting one region and undersculpting the adjacent region, which may result in a less than desirable final result.

In most patients, the upper approximately one-half of the lateral thigh is the region of most predominant deformity, so that deep sculpting is required in this area. The density of the adipose layer varies greatly from patient to patient. In individuals who have very dense fatty layers, use of a 3-mm Pinto cannula is helpful, beginning with the 15 cm length and then completing suctioning with the 20 cm length. Suctioning is done at midplane to deep plane. It is very important, especially in the initial phases of suctioning, to remain relatively deep in the fatty plane. At the midplane depth, I utilize a Cook cannula, usually 30 cm 3 mm, sculpting the entire length of the lateral thigh at midplane. To debulk and remove the additional fatty tissue, I switch to a 12-inch 10-gauge Klein cannula that will sculpt and smooth the entire lateral thigh. Finally, I finish the lateral thigh with a 12-inch 12-gauge Klein cannula, suctioning in a more superficial plane so as to remove surface irregularities and produce the final contour desired.

Surgical Procedure for the Medial Thighs and Knees

In individuals who do not require treatment of the anterior thighs, the posterior bulge of the medial thigh and the medial knee fat pad of the opposite leg may be treated at this time from the lateral decubitus position. As noted previously, if circumferential sculpting of the thighs is required, the medial thighs are best treated in a separate procedure, at the same time as the anterior thighs and knees (see Chapter 13).

At this point in the surgery, I turn the patient to the other side and repeat the process just described, treating the lateral flank, posterior flank, lateral thigh, posterior bulge of the medial thigh, and medial knee, if indicated. I then perform the sculpting of the buttocks, and, if necessary, the posterior thighs, from the prone position as described below. After suctioning of the buttocks and posterior thighs is completed, the patient is turned to the supine position to finish the treatment of the remaining anterior bulge of the medial thighs and infrapatellar fat pads. (See Chapter 13 for a complete description of the treatment of the medial thighs and knees.)

Surgical Procedure for the Buttocks

After treatment of both legs, the patient is placed in the prone position. A pillow is utilized for support directly under the pelvis, so that the buttocks are elevated. This permits the surgeon to sculpt the region effectively while maintaining its natural curves and producing a good blending between the buttocks, lateral thighs, and flank areas.

Sculpting is begun through the midline infragluteal crease incision, utilizing a 4-inch 12-gauge Klein spatula-type cannula in the midplane. The whole width of the buttock can be treated; however, the medial one-third of the buttock in its inferior one-third contains very soft fatty tissue, so that care must be taken not to overresect this area.

After sculpting the inferior one-third of the buttock, a 3-mm 15-cm Pinto cannula is utilized to suction in the deep plane. This deep suctioning effectively debulks the buttock. While advancing the cannula, one should lift and sculpt with the natural curve of the buttock, so as to retain this natural gently sloping curve, which gives the buttock its desirable cosmetic appearance. If a substantial amount of deep fat is present, a 3.5-mm Pinto cannula can also be utilized at this time.

After this, additional volume reduction is achieved in the deeper planes. I use a 3.0-mm or 3.5-mm Cook cannula measuring 30 or 35 cm in length to suction from the infragluteal crease incision up through the transition plane between the buttock and the posterior flank, effectively feathering the area to try to avoid any abrupt shelf in this region. If superficial irregularities and/or so-called cellulite are present, a 10-inch 12-gauge Klein cannula can be utilized for more superficial liposculpture at this point. I do not suction too superficially. One must remember that the infragluteal crease provides a strong point of support for the buttock, so that care should be made not to disturb its points of contact.

I do not recommend suctioning the buttocks from the lateral thigh incisions. Suctioning from this direction may tend to flatten the normal curvature of the buttock. If there is a large amount of thickening in the upper one-third of the buttock, suctioning can be done from the presacral incision on a lateral basis, angling down into the buttock. However, once again, this should be done conservatively. The goal is just to reduce this upper one-third volume and to feather between the buttocks and the posterior flank.

Surgical Procedure for the Posterior Thighs

A detailed description of liposculpture of the posterior thighs is presented in Chapter 12. The following is a summary of that procedure for continuity with the current procedure.

If the patient's lipodystrophy from the lateral thigh carries significantly onto the posterior thigh, and/or the posterior thigh is very lipodystrophic, it is advantageous to sculpt the posterior thigh at this time. Because the adjacent areas have already been tumesced, only a small additional amount of tumescent solution is required to completely anesthetize this area. Sculpting the posterior thigh additionally reduces the circumferential diameter of the thigh, produces a much improved cosmetic appearance, and may reduce the superficial irregularities (so-called cellulite) that are very common in this region.

Sculpting is begun on the posterior thigh through the infragluteal crease incision. In individuals who have excess adiposity only in the upper one-third of the posterior thigh, the so-called "banana roll" region, sculpting is done with a 4-inch 12-gauge Klein cannula. I try not to suction too deep or too superficially in this area, for this region is vital to the support of the buttocks. Excess suctioning of this upper one-third of the posterior thigh region may lead to ptosis of the buttocks.

At this point, I verify that there is good continuity and flow between the posterior thigh and lateral thigh. Any additional sculpting needed to ensure this smooth flow is done using the infragluteal crease incision.

By this point in time, the upper one-third of the posterior thigh will have already received adequate suctioning. Therefore, I begin suctioning below this point through the infragluteal crease incision, starting with a 6-inch 10-gauge and then a 10-inch 10-gauge Klein spatula-type cannula.

Then an inferior approach is taken through the posterior medial knee incision. One should not try to achieve all of the suctioning from the superior incision, for this may lead to overresection of the inferior gluteal crease. The inferior incision also provides good drainage for all areas, which are thoroughly interconnected by this point of the surgery. I begin with a 4-inch 12-gauge Klein spatula cannula, followed by a 6-inch 10-gauge and then 10-inch 10-gauge Klein spatula cannula. These cannulas, used deeply above the hamstring musculature, can reduce the volume and help produce a very desirable smooth effect to this region.

Then I generally utilize a 3.5-mm or 4-mm Cook cannula deeply on the fascia wall, suctioning the lower two-thirds of the posterior thigh. This is followed by a 12-inch 10-gauge Klein cannula and finally a 12-inch 12-gauge Klein cannula to complete the suctioning. Using the variety of cannulas may produce good volume reduction and good smoothing. Completing the suctioning on the relatively superficial plane with a spatula cannula can help to reduce many of the superficial surface irregularities that are present in this region.

After treatment of the buttocks and posterior thighs is completed, the lateral wedge protrusion, located superior and inferior to the lateral gluteal crease, is suctioned from the infragluteal crease incision. Then the patient is turned to the supine position to complete the treatment of the anterior bulge of the medial thighs and infrapatellar fat pads, as described in Chapter 13.

▷ Postoperative Considerations

The incision sites are cleaned and covered with absorbent pads. The patient is then fitted with a firm compression garment (Fig. 11-6), either above or below the knees, depending on whether the knees were included in the surgical procedure. This garment is left in place for approximately 12 hours postoperatively. For the first 24 to 48 hours, an absorbent undergarment may also be worn, if desired, to absorb the excess tumescent solution as it drains from the incisions.

For the remainder of the day of surgery, it is recommended that the patient rest, drink plenty of fluids, and eat light meals. The absorbent dressings may be slipped out and changed if they become saturated, but the surgical garment should be left in place.

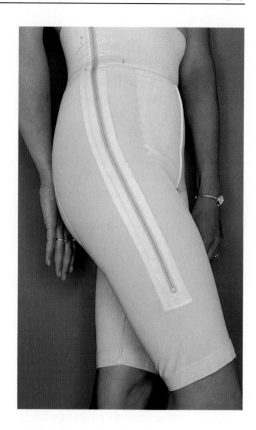

Figure 11-6
Patient wearing above-the-knee surgical garment following liposculpture of the buttocks, flanks, posterior thighs, medial thighs, and lateral thighs.

On the morning after the surgery, the patient may remove the garment and take a shower. When the the garment is removed, he or she should be well hydrated, and a companion should be present in case the patient becomes lightheaded from the release of the compression. Patients may shower as often as they like postoperatively, but no water immersion is permitted, either in the bathtub, hot tub, or swimming pool, until all the incisions have closed.

After showering, the patient should put on a clean dry compression garment with dry absorbent pads in place. Because the incision sites are not closed, drainage may be significant for the first 1 to 2 days. Thereafter, drainage is generally limited to the inferior incision sites, and a small gauze pad over those sites will usually absorb any excess solution.

Patients will progress with ambulation and activity as much as possible, beginning with the average patient taking a 2-mile walk on the first full postoperative day. The garment should be worn for 12 to 23 hours per day for the first postoperative week. After that, patients are told to electively wear the garment as they see fit. Because of the comfort level it provides, most patients will elect to wear the garment for an average of 2 to 3 weeks postoperatively. Patients are advised to stop the garment at their own discretion when it no longer feels beneficial.

Surgical compression hosiery, 20 to 30 mm pressure, in the form of panty hose may be helpful for patients who must be on their feet for long periods of time.

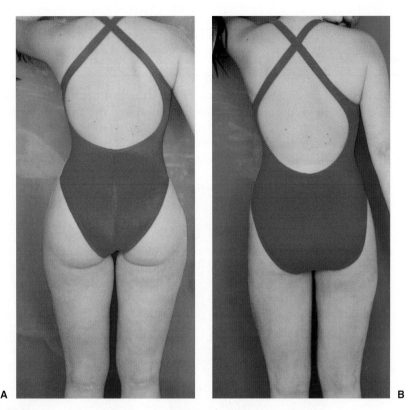

Figure 11-7

Female patient (**A**) before and (**B**) after liposculpture surgery of the flanks, buttocks, medial thighs, lateral thighs, posterior thighs, and knees.

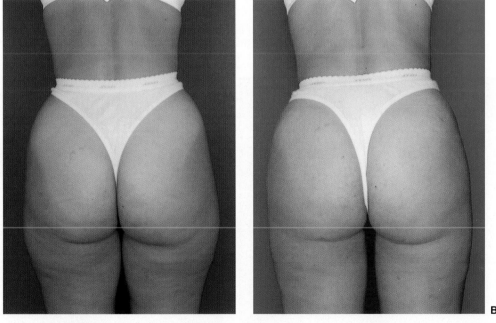

Figure 11-8

Female patient (**A**) before and (**B**) after liposculpture surgery of the flanks, buttocks, lateral thighs, medial thighs, and posterior thighs. Note reduction in "cellulite."

▷ Results

Postoperatively (Figs. 11-7 to 11-11), the buttocks, hips, and thighs are smaller overall, with a smoother flowing line over the hips, a more natural-looking "lifted" buttock, and the reduction of banana rolls, saddlebags, and other bulges or fatty accumulations. The body achieves a more symmetrical appearance after Three-Dimensional Tumescent Liposculpture™.

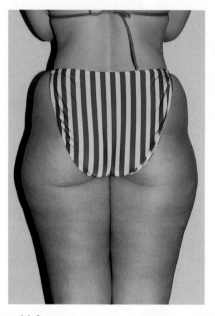
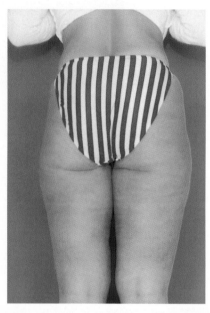

A   B

Figure 11-9

Female patient (**A**) before and (**B**) after liposculpture surgery of the flanks, buttocks, medial thighs, lateral thighs, and posterior thighs. Note "violin" deformity preoperatively, caused by the lateral gluteal depression.

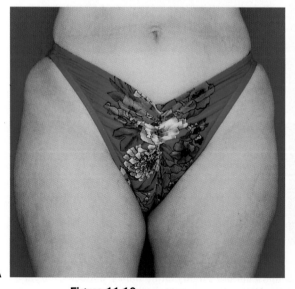
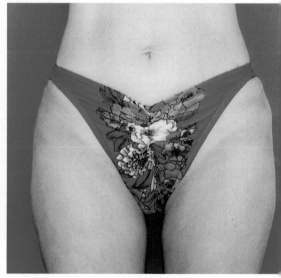

A

Figure 11-10

Female patient (**A**) before and (**B**) after liposculpture surgery of the flanks, buttocks, medial thighs, and lateral thighs.

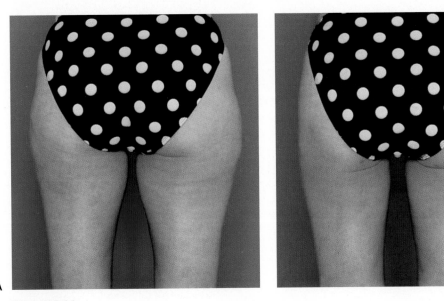

A   B

Figure 11-11
Female patient (**A**) before and (**B**) after liposculpture surgery of the flanks, buttocks, medial thighs, lateral thighs, and posterior thighs.

CHAPTER 12

LIPOSCULPTURE OF THE POSTERIOR THIGHS

Preoperative Evaluation ▶ *Surgical Procedure* ▶ *Postoperative Considerations*

The posterior thigh is an interesting anatomic area that is too often neglected by surgeons. In the early days of liposuction technology, the posterior thigh was a difficult area to treat. However, the development of smaller cannulas made it possible to achieve much better results in this area.

The posterior thighs often exhibit multiple superficial irregularities (so-called "cellulite"), which make the site very disfiguring for women, especially in short shorts or bathing suits. (See Chapter 13 for a more extensive discussion of this condition.) No matter how well one contours the lateral and medial thighs, if the posterior thighs protrude irregularly and show multiple skin irregularities, the patient's degree of satisfaction may be lessened. A much better cosmetic result can be achieved through a coordinated treatment of the lateral, posterior, and medial thighs.

Treatment of the thighs may need to be carried out in several separate surgical procedures. I seldom contour around the entire thigh during a single treatment session because this often causes significant postoperative swelling and a much more extended recovery time. The postoperative edema of the ankles may be slow to resolve if the lymphatic drainage from the lower extremity has been compromised by full-circumference surgery. The swelling is less pronounced and resolves much more promptly when at least 25% of the thigh is left untreated, to carry the lymphatic drainage from the lower extremity.

In keeping with the concept of Three-Dimensional Tumescent Liposculpture™, the posterior thighs should not be considered in isolation. The entire anatomic area, including the buttocks and the upper legs, should be evaluated as a unit, and one or more procedures should be planned to achieve the desired results.

121

▷ Preoperative Evaluation

A thorough preoperative evaluation and a careful explanation of realistic expectations are crucial in treating the posterior thighs. Generally, I tell my patients that I cannot eradicate cellulite. In actual clinical practice, I can often eliminate many of the posterior thigh irregularities with careful treatment, using small cannulas in a relatively superficial fashion. If patients approach the procedure with decreased expectations, they tend to be very pleased when they find that the areas of dimpling have been reduced. However, patient satisfaction in this case is very much a matter of expectation. If they expect liposculpture to get rid of all the cellulite, which is nearly impossible with any type of treatment, they may be dissatisfied even with a substantial cosmetic improvement in the area.

During the preoperative evaluation, it is important to take note of the status of the venous circulation and the number of varicosities in the area. If the patient has large varicosities, reducing the fatty component of this region may have the effect of making the varicosities even more pronounced. If the patient's venous circulation is poor, then a greater than usual amount of ecchymosis may result postoperatively.

Care must be taken in treating the posterior thigh. The upper portion of the posterior thigh tends, in some individuals, to be very prominent. This so-called "banana roll" area must be treated with great caution, because this is one of the anatomic features that maintains the position of the buttocks, along with the suspensory fibers of the infragluteal crease. Overzealous sculpting in this area may leave a depression in the region, which is unsightly and cosmetically unacceptable, and may also lead to ptosis of the buttocks.

Aside from these cautions, the posterior thigh area tends to be "user-friendly." When it is treated along with the adjacent lateral and medial thighs and the knees, if necessary, one can achieve excellent results in this region (see Figs. 11-7 to 11-11).

▷ Surgical Procedure

The operative areas are marked with a gentian violet pen with the patient in the standing position (Figs. 12-1, 12-2).

The posterior thigh region is usually approached through two incisions, one in the mid-infragluteal crease, the other on the inferior medial portion of the thigh adjacent to the medial knee fat pad, called the posterior medial knee incision, which can also be used to access the medial knee fat pad if desired.

The patient is placed in the prone position with a pillow under the pelvis. Sculpting is begun through the infragluteal crease incision with a 4-inch 12-gauge Klein spatula cannula. This sculpting should be done in midplane so as not to be too superficial, but also not so deep as to remove the supporting mechanisms, which will lead to the above-mentioned ptosis of the buttocks. Careful sculpting from the infragluteal incision will reduce the size of the banana roll of adiposity in this infragluteal region.

At this point, I verify that there is good continuity and flow between the pos-

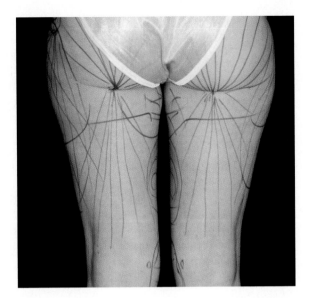

Figure 12-1

Preoperative markings for liposculpture surgery of the buttocks, posterior thighs, medial thighs, lateral thighs, and knees. Note concentric circles at mid-medial thigh in area of depression.

terior thigh and lateral thigh. Any additional sculpting needed to ensure this smooth flow is done using the infragluteal crease incision.

By this point in time, the upper one-third of the posterior thigh will have already received adequate suctioning. Therefore, I begin suctioning below this point through the infragluteal crease incision, starting with a 6-inch 10-gauge and then a 10-inch 10-gauge Klein cannula.

Next, the inferior incision is utilized, beginning with a 4-inch 12-gauge Klein spatula cannula, increasing to a 6-inch 10-gauge and then a 10-inch 10-gauge

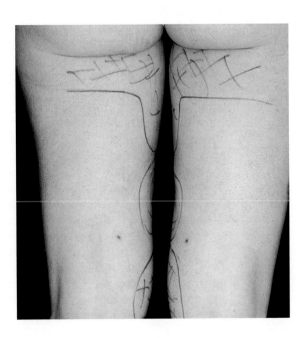

Figure 12-2

Preoperative markings for liposculpture surgery of the "banana roll," medial thighs, and knees.

Klein cannula. In most individuals, this sequence of cannulas will effectively cover the lower two-thirds of the posterior thigh region. It is important to approach the area from the inferior position so as not to oversuction in the upper one-third of the thigh, which may lead to less acceptable cosmetic results.

After the inferior suctioning, I return to the superior midline infragluteal incision and sculpt with a 3.5-mm Cook cannula 30 or 35 cm in length. This sculpting should be done deep, close to the hamstring musculature overriding the fascial plane, so as to achieve a good reduction in the mass of adiposity in this area.

Attention is then given to the superficial irregularities. I use a 12-inch 12-gauge Klein cannula to help reduce the superficial irregularities and smooth the area.

The above approach gives both deep and superficial suctioning to an area that, if left untreated, may detract from the rest of the sculpting of the lateral and medial thigh. The area is especially important to many patients because of the superficial irregularities and dimpling, called cellulite, which commonly occur in that region.

▷ Postoperative Considerations

Following the procedure, the incision sites are dressed in the usual fashion. A below-the-knee surgical garment is put on to ensure good compression to the site. This is especially important if the medial knee region has been treated concurrently.

The patient should rest for the remainder of the surgical day and maintain good hydration. The garment should be left in place until the next morning. If the absorbent pads become too moist, they can be slipped out and clean dry pads inserted. If drainage is heavy, the patient may also wish to wear an absorbent undergarment.

In the morning, the garment and pads are carefully removed and the patient should take a shower. After showering, a clean surgical garment is put on with absorbent pads in place.

Immediate ambulation is encouraged, with a 2-mile walk suggested for most patients the day after surgery. Recovery is much more rapid if the patient ambulates as much as possible immediately after the surgery, especially when the lower extremities are treated.

In addition to walking, the patient may begin exercises on the second postoperative day. On subsequent days, stair-stepping exercises provide the most benefit to the patient, giving good contraction of the quadriceps, hamstring, and buttocks muscles, and reducing the postoperative tissue edema. The exercises do not need to be carried out rapidly; it is the mere repetitive motion that is beneficial. After exercise, periodic elevation of the legs may be helpful to reduce swelling and provide the patient with greater comfort.

Generally, patients will wear the surgical garment 12 to 23 hours the first day and then electively as they see fit. Most patients choose to wear the garment half-time for 2 to 3 weeks. If the patient wears the garment during sleeping hours, the legs should not be elevated in bed. Prolonged elevation of the legs while wearing the compression garment may compromise the blood supply to the area.

Patients who must stand at their job for long periods of time may wish to wear surgical compression hosiery, 20 to 30 mm, in the form of panty hose. This is especially helpful for individuals such as flight attendants, who are not only on their feet a great deal, but also have pressure effects from the aircraft. The hosiery may be continued for as long as it gives the patient comfort. Again, it should not be worn at night, or if it is, the legs should not be elevated.

CHAPTER 13

LIPOSCULPTURE OF THE ANTERIOR THIGHS, MEDIAL THIGHS, AND KNEES

Surgical Procedure ▶ *Postoperative Considerations* ▶ *Results*

The anterior thighs, medial thighs, and knees constitute an important area for liposculpture and should be considered as a three-dimensional cosmetic unit. The surgeon will often encounter individuals who have very full thighs, despite having a very slim upper body and small waist. The thighs may be treated in one procedure or two, depending on the extent of the lipodystrophic changes.

When the patient has lipodystrophy in the area overlying the quadriceps muscle, the changes generally blend into the medial thighs and the knee areas, so that this entire area may be treated in a single procedure. If the patient requires liposculpture of the entire circumferential thigh, this unit would represent the second step in a two-step process.

In my experience, attempts to circumferentially sculpt the entire thigh in one surgical procedure may produce inferior results. The surgical procedure itself is limited by the amount of tumescent solution that can be infiltrated at one time. In addition, procedures that involve the entire circumference of the thigh tend to have significant postoperative swelling. When the thigh is treated in two stages, the patient experiences more uniform contouring and better postoperative recovery. The first stage, described in Chapter 11, usually includes the lateral and posterior flanks, the lateral thighs, the buttocks, and either the upper posterior thighs or the entire posterior thighs, depending on the degree of lipodystrophic change that is present. After a period of 2 or more weeks, a second procedure may be performed to sculpt the anterior thighs, medial thighs, and knees, as described in this chapter. If desired, the calves may also be included in this procedure (see Chapter 14 for a description of liposculpture of the calves).

Preoperatively, the patient must be carefully counseled as to realistic expectations that can be achieved. Patients often have the most unrealistic expectations as to final achievable results in this area, so that proper patient selection is extremely important. There are a number of limiting factors that will determine the exact degree of sculpting possible and the amount of balance one will be able to achieve between upper and lower body symmetry.

The first limiting factor is the relative size of the underlying musculature. Many individuals have highly developed quadriceps and hamstring muscles and a very large muscular component to their lower extremities. In addition to the muscular component, they frequently have lipodystrophic changes overlying the anterior and posterior compartments. The surgeon is able to balance and sculpt the thigh compartments, but the musculature obviously will remain intact. Postoperatively, if the patient pursues a moderate exercise program and achieves a modest weight loss, some of this bulk can be reduced. However, genetic considerations and body type will be the limiting factors in many individuals. Other individuals have poorly developed quadriceps musculature with increased amounts of adipose tissue in the anterior thigh. A high degree of exercise postoperatively will help reduce swelling and improve the contour of the anterior thigh.

The second important factor to consider is the patient's skin elasticity. The procedure of liposculpture may, when performed correctly, help tighten the overlying skin, and with a well-chosen postoperative exercise program patients may achieve good skin tightening in most cases. However, the extent of skin laxity must be evaluated and discussed preoperatively, so that patients have realistic expectations about what can be achieved and understand the importance of postoperative exercise.

The third factor is the presence of compartmentalized fat, or so-called "cellulite," especially in the anterior thigh region. This cellulite results from attachment of the skin to the underlying muscular fascia in such a manner that the angles of attachment form alternating areas of depression and protrusion, with the areas of protrusion containing regions of hypertrophic fat. This causes an irregular or dimpled appearance to the skin. Most clinicians consider these changes in the skin to be a genetic tendency and probably a normal variant. However, patients consider cellulite an unsightly disorder. A variety of creams and other therapies were tried to remedy this situation, but all were relatively ineffective until relatively superficial liposuction with small cannulas became available. This technique permits the surgeon to eliminate some, but usually not all, of the cellulite. By careful use of small cannulas near the surface, attachment of the septal bands, which cause the depressed areas, can be carefully released and the superficial protruding fat removed. This combined effect results in a smoothing of the surface into a much more satisfactory cosmetic appearance. A realistic approach preoperatively is to advise the patient that the surgeon's ability to remove cellulite is limited, and not to promise any significant improvement. When improvement often does occur, patients are typically very grateful and tend to be pleased with the greater than expected improvement in their appearance.

▷ Surgical Procedure

The operative areas are marked with a gentian violet pen with the patient in the standing position (Figs. 13-1 to 13-3).

Generally, the anterior and medial thighs and knees require a larger volume of tumescent solution than one might anticipate and a longer time to suction completely than might be expected. However, the areas do not tend to be as sensitive as some other regions, so that a solution containing 0.05% lidocaine is usually adequate for the anterior thigh compartment, with a 0.1% concentration of lidocaine being utilized for the medial thigh and knee areas. This initial anesthesia can be reinforced by a small amount of 0.1% lidocaine solution to the anterior compartment just prior to surgery.

The anterior thigh is usually accessed through incisions on the lateral and medial knee fold and the superior lateral thigh. The medial thigh is accessed through a lateral pubic incision and also an incision in the infragluteal crease. The knees are accessed by the same medial knee fold incision as that used for the anterior thigh, as well as an inferior medial knee incision at the lowermost portion of the lipodystrophy overlying the medial knee. The medial and lateral infrapatellar fat pads are accessed by small incisions adjacent to the fat pads themselves.

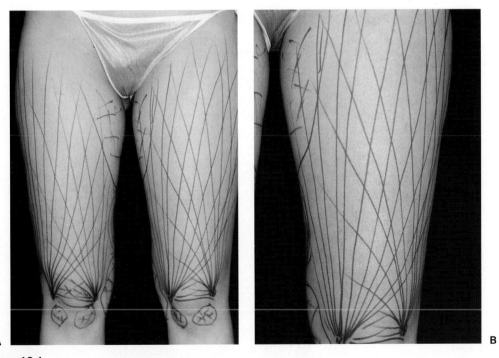

A   B

Figure 13-1

A, B: Preoperative markings for liposculpture surgery of the anterior thighs, medial thighs, and knees.

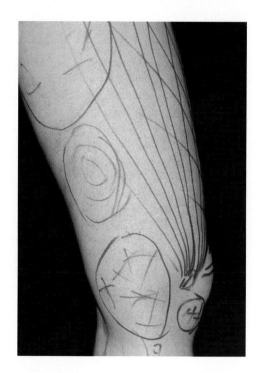

Figure 13-2
Preoperative markings for liposculpture surgery of the anterior thighs, medial thighs, and knees. Note midmedial thigh depression, marked with concentric circles; this area will not be suctioned.

Surgical Procedure for the Anterior Thighs

I begin this cosmetic unit of surgery by treating the anterior thigh. The anterior thigh can be one of the most challenging areas of the body to sculpt so as to produce a uniform smooth appearance of the surface. It is very important to stay in the midplane and deep plane. Extensive superficial liposculpture in the anterior thigh area may lead to rippling and irregularities, which may be difficult to correct. It is also important to allow adequate time to sculpt this area. I spend as

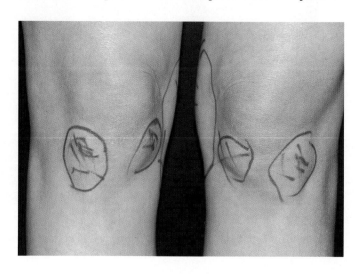

Figure 13-3
Preoperative markings for liposculpture surgery of the medial knees and infrapatellar fat pads.

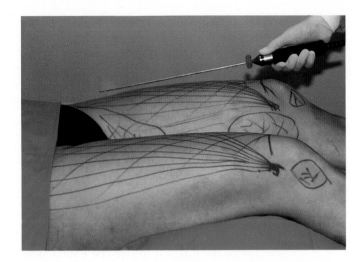

Figure 13-4

Supine position of the patient for liposculpture of the anterior thighs from the knee fold incision.

much time sculpting the anterior thighs, medial thighs, and knees as I do on the lateral and posterior flanks; buttocks; and lateral, posterior, and medial thighs.

The patient is placed in the supine position with a pillow under the knees for this procedure. The anterior thigh is suctioned by alternating between the medial and lateral knee fold incisions (Fig. 13-4). First, I use a 4-inch Klein spatula cannula, either 12- or 14-gauge, to carefully sculpt the fat in the suprapatellar region. This area tends to be a very fibrofatty region. With time and gravity this area tends to become quite ptotic, producing a bulge that protrudes at, or slightly below, the superior aspect of the patella. The patient perceives this as a cosmetic deformity, so it is very important to treat this area adequately.

After the suprapatellar area has been sculpted, the rest of the anterior thigh is treated. I use a 12-gauge Klein spatula cannula in progressively increasing lengths, first 6 inch, then 10 inch, and finally 12 inch, alternating between the lateral and medial knee fold incisions so as to form a crisscrossing pattern over the entire surface of the anterior thigh. With each stroke, the cannula is moved over approximately 1 cm, so that a uniform sculpting can be achieved from lateral to medial or medial to lateral, depending on the point of entry. This area must be treated with great care, being careful not to suction too superficially.

I then change to a 3-mm Cook cannula 30 or 35 cm in length, which is a user-friendly cannula for treating this area. Its open-ended nature allows good removal of the fat but, because its end openings are all on the inferior half of the cannula, it tends to reduce tunneling into the dermis. This allows enough of the small subcutaneous fat pad to remain so that the area will have a smooth surface on completion of the sculpting. For patients who have extensive thickness of the fat pad, a 3.5- or 4-mm Cook cannula may be utilized to additionally debulk the area.

Next, the superior lateral thigh incision is utilized to additionally sculpt the thickest aspect of the anterior thigh fat pad, which usually lies in the upper one-third of the fatty compartment overlying the quadriceps muscle. This approach allows good crisscrossing of this area as well as debulking to produce an overall thinning effect of the anterior thigh compartment. I use 14- and 12-gauge Klein spatula cannulas, 6 or 10 inches in length, as well as a 3-mm 30-cm Cook cannula for this area.

Next, I utilize the lateral and medial knee fold incisions for medium depth suctioning with a 12-inch 10-gauge Klein spatula cannula, again crisscrossing the area. Suctioning is then completed through these incisions with a 12-inch 12-gauge Klein cannula, which can be used relatively superficially at this time so as to treat any areas of compartmentalization or so-called cellulite changes. This must be done carefully and not too aggressively, so as to retain an adequate amount of superficial fat to leave the area as smooth as possible.

Surgical Procedure for the Knees

The knees are treated next, with the patient still in the supine position with a pillow under the knees. I utilize the medial knee fold incision to sculpt the lipodystrophic area on the medial knee as well as the adjacent medial infrapatellar fat pad. These areas are treated using a combination of 4-inch 12-gauge Klein cannulas and 4-inch 11-gauge Cook cannulas. Access is made from the medial knee fold incision and the inferior medial knee incision to obtain good crisscrossing of the areas. Fairly definitive removal of the fat in the medial area can be performed to reduce this fat pad as much as possible.

On the superior aspect of the medial knee fat pad, one must take care to transition this area into the middle one-third of the medial thigh region. This area is commonly very thin and, to achieve a better overall appearance of the medial thigh and knee axis, little or no suctioning should be done in this area. If one oversuctions this middle one-third, the patient may be left with a persistent bow-legged appearance of the leg, which results from a pronounced upper medial thigh fat pad and medial knee fat pads.

If lipodystrophy extends down onto the medial aspect of the calf or shin, careful blending should be continued into this area, to effect good contouring of the entire region.

The lateral infrapatellar fat pad is also accessed through the lateral knee fold incision. It should be treated with 14- and 12-gauge 4-inch Klein cannulas and the 4-inch 11-gauge Cook cannula. If one fails to treat these infrapatellar fat pads, the patient may be left with the appearance of so-called "housemaid knees." This may negate the positive effect produced by suctioning the medial knee fat pad.

Surgical Procedure for the Medial Thighs

The area of lipodystrophy in the upper one-third of the medial thigh is next treated. If the cosmetic unit being treated includes the anterior thighs, medial thighs, and knees, the patient will be in the supine position at this point. In this case, the anterior bulge of the medial thighs is treated first, followed by the posterior bulge of the medial thigh from the lateral decubitus position. However, if the cosmetic unit being treated includes the lateral and posterior flanks, buttocks, lateral thighs, medial thighs and posterior thighs, the patient is in the lateral de-cubitus position at this point, and the posterior bulge of the medial thigh is treated first. The posterior bulge encompasses about 70% of the medial thigh and the an-terior bulge about 30%.

Posterior Bulge of the Medial Thighs

With the patient in the lateral decubitus position with the top leg drawn forward, the medial thigh of the bottom leg is ideally exposed for treatment (see Fig. 11-5). I begin sculpting the medial thigh of the bottom leg using the infragluteal crease incision. To avoid overresecting the "banana roll" area, I divide it into two halves, lateral and medial, with the midpoint at the infragluteal crease incision. During liposculpture of the medial thigh, I suction only the medial half of the ba-nana roll. I leave the lateral half of the banana roll untouched at this time if it is included in the cosmetic unit and will be suctioned later. However, if the cosmetic unit being treated is the anterior thigh, medial thigh, and knees, I will not be suc-tioning the banana roll later. In that case, I feather into the lateral banana roll when the patient is turned on the other side.

I begin treatment with a 4-inch 12-gauge Klein cannula. Next I switch to a 10-gauge Klein cannula, first 6 inches and then 10 inches in length. Sculpting is done in midplane, being careful not to sculpt too superficially in this area. Then I use a 25-cm Cook cannula, either 3 or 3.5 mm, in the deep plane. It is important to be very methodical and focused during this suctioning, and to carefully move the cannula in a progressive fashion along the plane to be resected. Because the adipose layer in this region is very soft, it is easy to overresect, which may lead to undesirable results that are difficult to repair.

Following use of the Cook cannula, I utilize a 10-inch 10-gauge Klein spat-ula cannula midplane, and then a 10-inch 12-gauge Klein cannula slightly more superficially, to complete sculpting of the medial thigh from the lateral decubitus position. Again, only a limited number of passes should be made in this area. With the patient in this lateral decubitus position with the upper leg extended, a clear perspective view of the medial thigh is obtained, and one can palpate and visual-ize what the final result will be. Approximately 70% of the medial thigh resec-tioning is done through this posterior gluteal crease incision.

Anterior Bulge of the Medial Thighs

The remaining 30% of the medial thigh bulge is best approached through a lateral pubic incision with the patient in a supine position. This incision is made superior to the inguinal crease, 2 to 3 cm medial to the femoral pulse. One should avoid the inguinal crease itself, because this area may be slow to heal and in some indi-viduals may be prone to hypertrophic scarring. This incision superior to the in-guinal crease avoids any scars in the medial thigh area itself, which may be cos-metically unacceptable to the patient and may have a tendency to become exaggerated because of depression around the incision site.

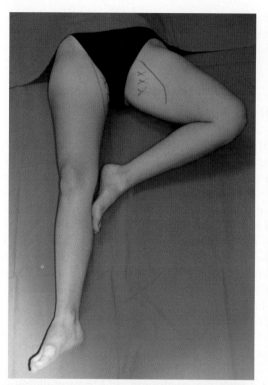

A

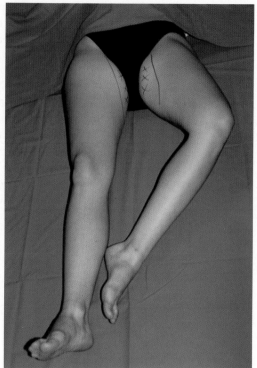

B

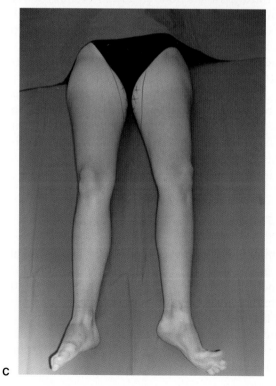

C

Figure 13-5

A: Patient in the full frogleg position; **B**: patient in the semi-frogleg position; **C**: patient in the fully extended position for suctioning of the anterior bulge of the medial thigh in the supine position.

In effect, I obtain three different angles of approach through this one incision by using three positions of the leg: the full frogleg position, the semi-frogleg position, and the fully extended position (Fig. 13-5). The full frogleg position is obtained by having the patient place the sole of one foot against the knee of the opposite leg and rotate the bent leg as far laterally as is comfortable. What I call the semi-frogleg position is the frog position reduced by one-half, with the sole of the foot placed against the calf of the opposite leg. The fully extended position consists of the leg being straightened with only slight outward rotation of the thigh. Use of these three positions allows good crisscrossing of the area while minimizing the number of surgical incisions.

The intent of suctioning through the lateral pubic incision is to remove approximately 30% of the fat pad that exists in the upper anterior bulge of the medial thigh region; this is the anteriormost fat pad of this region. The fat of this area tends to be quite soft and should be treated very carefully, with the surgeon remaining extremely focused to avoid oversuctioning. I treat one side at a time, starting with the patient positioned in the full frogleg position. I begin with a 4-inch 12-gauge Klein cannula. Then I use a 6-inch 10-gauge Klein cannula and then a 10-inch 10-gauge Klein cannula. The cannula should be carefully moved from lateral to medial, approximately 1 cm with each stroke, so that the fat pad is removed in a uniform fashion. Extreme care should be taken not to oversuction this region. Even a minimal number of passes of the cannula may result in over-sculpting of this area.

The semi-frogleg position is then utilized, which permits an additional direction of suctioning without changing the entry point. While continuously observing and palpating the area, several additional strokes may be taken with the 10-inch 10-gauge Klein cannula and then the 10-inch 12-gauge Klein cannula.

Finally, the leg is placed in the fully extended position, nearly straight with a slight outward rotation, and suctioning is completed using a 10-inch 12-gauge Klein cannula.

Because the majority of suctioning will have been performed from the infragluteal incision, this anterior approach primarily achieves removal of the bulge of adipose tissue that occurs, and is easily visible, when the person is in a sitting position. This bulge forms a less than desirable excess roll of fatty tissue adjacent to the groin fold. Caution is needed, however, because a hollow depression in this area from overresecting is equally as objectionable cosmetically.

▷ Postoperative Considerations

On completion of treatment, the areas are cleaned and dressed, and a below-the-knee compression garment is applied (Fig. 13-6). This garment should be worn continuously overnight. If necessary, the absorbent pads may be slipped out from under it and dry pads positioned. Drainage from the excision sites may be significant, especially for the first 24 to 48 hours postoperatively.

Patients should rest at home for the remainder of that day, drinking plenty of fluids and eating light meals. The legs may be elevated from time to time but should not be elevated at night with the compression garment in place.

In the morning, patients will remove the surgical garment and take a shower.

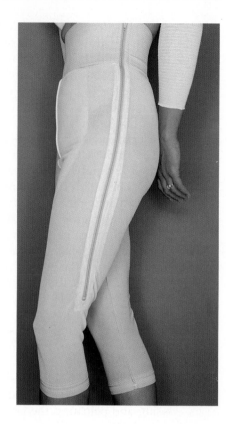

Figure 13-6

Patient wearing below-the-knee surgical garment following liposculpture of the anterior thighs, medial thighs, and knees.

A companion should be present because they may become light-headed when they first remove the compression garment. After showering, a clean compression garment is positioned over dry absorbent pads. During the postoperative period patients may shower as often as they like, but they should avoid any water immersion until all the incision sites have closed.

As with all of my liposculpture procedures, patients are immediately ambulatory, with a suggested 2-mile walk on the first postoperative day. The following day patients can resume more active exercise. Stepping exercises provide the best and fastest recovery after liposculpture of the anterior thighs. Movement of the underlying quadriceps muscle tends to milk the excessive solution and edema from this compartment and expedites the recovery. At a later time, more vigorous and active stair-stepping activities may also aid in the tightening of the skin over the medial and anterior thighs. Such exercises may produce superior results if done diligently, especially in the immediate postoperative period.

Compression hosiery, 20 to 30 mm in the form of a panty hose, is helpful for patients who must stand at their jobs for long periods of time. This is especially important for individuals such as flight attendants, who are not only on their feet a great deal but also suffer pressure effects from the aircraft. If patients elect to wear the panty hose, I suggest that they wear the compression garment with it. They may wish to continue using the compression hosiery for several months postoperatively, to aid in the recovery and reduce the amount of postoperative edema. I tell my patients that the anterior thighs stay swollen the longest period

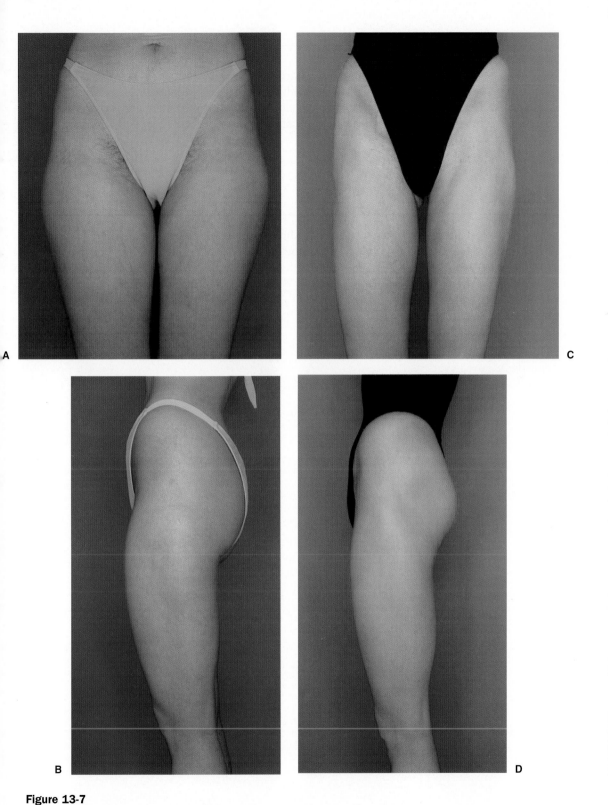

Figure 13-7

Female patient (**A,B**) before and (**C,D**) after liposculpture surgery in two stages. Stage I consisted of the lateral and posterior flanks, buttocks, lateral thighs, and posterior thighs; stage II consisted of the medial thighs, anterior thighs, and knees.

of time, and that the best results are seen 6 to 12 months postoperatively, especially in patients who continue a diligent exercise program.

Occasionally, edema may develop postoperatively after any surgery done in the thigh areas. A mild diuretic can be prescribed to reduce this postoperative edema.

▷ Results

Postoperatively, these patients show smaller appearing thighs, reduction of bulges, and a smoother flowing line from the groin to the knees (Fig. 13-7).

CHAPTER 14

LIPOSCULPTURE OF THE CALVES AND ANKLES

Preoperative Evaluation ▶ *Surgical Procedure* ▶ *Postoperative Care*

Liposculpture of the calves and ankles presents a challenge for the surgeon. This area requires excellent technique, good preoperative consultation and evaluation, and a very cooperative patient. I recommend that the surgeon have a good deal of experience in treating other body areas before attempting to sculpt the calves and ankles. This area may not be forgiving. The cosmetic disability in this area is caused by a relatively small amount of excess fat, and there is not much room for technical error.

However, liposculpture of the calves and ankles plays an important cosmetic role for the patient who has the so-called "piano leg" type of deformity. This deformity is present when the lower diameter of the calf at the ankle approaches the upper diameter of the calf, so that the leg does not have its normal tapered proportions. Such patients find it difficult to wear skirts and shorts without a high level of embarrassment. Liposculpture may greatly reduce or eliminate this cosmetic problem. Therefore, if done correctly in the proper patient, a high level of satisfaction may be achieved for the surgeon and the patient.

▷ Preoperative Evaluation

A careful history must be taken in order to determine the patient's predisposing factors. Of particular interest are extreme varicosities and any previous history of lymphedema. Generally, younger patients are the best candidates for this procedure. The patient should be evaluated for any significant number of varicosities

139

and should be questioned as to a history of edema, especially pitting edema, which may not be helped by the procedure and, in fact, may actually worsen as a result of the surgery.

The patient's bony and muscular configuration must be evaluated to determine the actual degree of improvement that one could realistically expect. Also, the adjacent knee areas should be evaluated. If liposculpture of the knees has not been previously performed or is indicated, the knees can be treated at the same time as the calves and ankles (see Chapter 13). The majority of fat is found in the posterior half of the calf and ankle area. There is very little fatty tissue in the pretibial and adjacent areas, so that suctioning of the anterior aspect of the leg is usually not necessary.

The patient's expectations regarding this surgery must be determined. Patients must be advised that, after the surgery, a good level of appropriate physical exercise will be required to expedite recovery, along with periodic elevation of the legs to provide good drainage of any swelling that might occur. Of utmost importance is that the patient must agree to wear good compression hosiery, in the range of 30 to 40 mm of pressure, usually for several months following the surgery. Normal store-bought support hosiery may not be adequate after this type of procedure. Depending on the age of the individual and the severity of the lipodystrophic areas that need to be treated, as well as the overall venous and lymphatic return in the area, this type of compression should be carried on for a matter of months. I usually advise patients to plan on wearing the compression hosiery for 3 to 6 months postoperatively. If recovery should proceed more rapidly, they will be able discontinue their use at an earlier date.

▷ Surgical Procedure

The operative sites are marked with a gentian violet pen (Fig. 14-1). Patients are asked to stand on their toes during marking. The lower border of the gastrocnemius muscle is identified and marked, so that attention can be given while sculpting to enhancing the definition of this anatomic landmark.

Generally, for the calves and ankles I use six incisions on each leg: one on each side of the ankle, one on each side of the midcalf, and one on each side of the superior aspect of the calf. Crisscrossing is achieved from the medial and lateral incisions, so that very precise reduction of the fatty layer is achieved. One must be cautious not to suction too superficially, because any irregularity or grooving that might result in this area may be difficult to improve and may leave a less satisfactory cosmetic appearance.

I generally use a tumescent solution containing 0.1% lidocaine for this area (see Chapter 5).

The patient is placed in the prone position, with a foam pillow under the pretibial area so that the incisions at the ankles can be easily accessed. I begin suctioning with a 4-inch 12-gauge Klein spatula cannula, which allows a precise contouring around the Achilles tendon and the ankle area. Then I increase to a 6-inch and then a 10-inch 12-gauge Klein spatula cannula. This type of cannula is user-friendly, neither too small nor too large, and generally gives a good smooth sur-

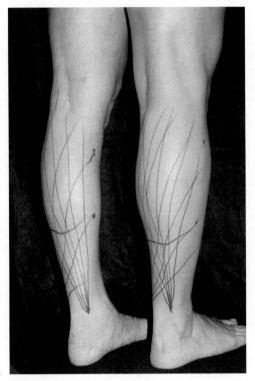
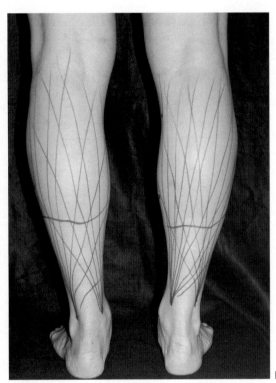

Figure 14-1

A,B: Preoperative markings for liposculpture surgery of the calves and ankles.

face contour. In general, the longer cannulas give the surgeon the advantage of good stroke areas for treating the entire cosmetic unit, while the shorter cannulas provide better control.

Next, I suction through the midcalf incisions to additionally contour upward and downward on the calf fat pad. I utilize 6-inch and 10-inch 12-gauge Klein spatula cannulas for this suctioning. I then suction the calf downward from the superior incisions with the same cannulas.

The knees can be treated at this time if they are to be included in this surgical procedure. (See Chapter 13 for a discussion of liposculpture of the knees.)

Depending on the thickness of the fat pad, I then suction through the ankle incisions and the midcalf incision, using a 3-mm Cook cannula, either 30 or 35 cm length, depending on the amount of lipodystrophy present and the size of the calf. Staying deep will remove the remainder of the excess adipose tissue in the calf regions. After this, I return to the 10- or 12-inch 12-gauge Klein spatula cannula to complete suctioning, so as to achieve good blending and smoothing of the surface. It is important to attempt to obtain good definition around the Achilles tendon and around the lower border of the gastrocnemius muscle.

To determine the end point, one can easily visualize and palpate the changes in the fatty layer in this area. It is important to attempt not to oversuction this anatomic region.

▷ Postoperative Care

At the conclusion of the operation, the incision sites are cleaned and covered with absorbent dressings. Patients are then fitted with good quality compression hose such as Jobst compression stockings (see Appendix), 30 to 40 mm pressure. They should wear these compression stockings for at least 3 weeks. Some patients will need to wear them for 3 to 6 months. In the immediate postoperative period, it is a good idea for the patients to wear the compression stockings even while in bed at night, with the legs at a horizontal plane or very minimally elevated. With these highly compressive stockings, any significant elevation at night should be avoided, because it might compromise the arterial blood supply if the elevation persists for long periods of time.

Patients should rest for the remainder of the day of surgery, drinking plenty of fluids and eating light meals. The next day they should shower and then take a 2-mile walk. Early ambulation is important in recovering from any liposculpture to the leg areas. The legs should be elevated after exercise and periodically throughout the day.

On the second day after surgery, patients may return to work and gradually resume normal activities. If they have a sedentary job or one that requires constant standing, it is recommended that they take breaks to permit periods of leg elevation and/or ambulation.

Postoperative exercise is very important. Exercises using a stationary bicycle or stair-stepper are particularly helpful. Any transient edema can be treated with a diuretic such as hydrochlorothiazide/triamterene (Dyazide). This is especially helpful for patients who are on their feet a lot or are sedentary in their work.

CHAPTER 15

LIPOSCULPTURE OF THE ARMS, AXILLARY FOLDS, AND DOWAGER'S HUMP

Preoperative Evaluation ▶ *Surgical Procedure* ▶ *Postoperative Considerations* ▶ *Results*

The arms constitute an important anatomic site for liposculpture. The primary area of excess adipose accumulation is in the posterior aspect of the upper arm overlying the triceps musculature. If there is fullness in the anterior and posterior axillary folds, they may also be treated at this time. If the infrascapular fat pad has not been included in previous surgical procedures, it may be included with this procedure as well, to complete the three-dimensional approach and achieve circumferential liposculpture.

The upper arms are important to the overall appearance, particularly in women who like to wear short-sleeved or sleeveless clothing, making this area cosmetically conspicuous. There is a strong psychological overlay to flabby arms for the female psyche. Nowadays, when many women desire a high level of fitness, a hanging or flabby appearance of the arms is undesirable. Also, the fashion industry currently emphasizes broader shoulders, thinner arms, and a fuller upper body appearance in an effort to better proportionalize the relative size of the hips and thighs.

Liposculpture can be performed on the posterior arm without difficulty. In the majority of cases, one simple incision just above the elbow is sufficient to achieve the desired contouring. In my experience, it has never been necessary to excise any excess skin from the arms.

In most cases, the surgeon is able to develop a much more youthful, lean appearance, with good tapering of the arm from the axilla to the elbow. Patient satisfaction after the procedure is quite high, provided that the patient was a suitable candidate to begin with and had appropriate expectations. For a good final result, it is important that patients be willing to do some form of simple arm exercises postoperatively that emphasize skin contracture over the triceps muscle. This area tends to be underdeveloped by normal day-to-day activities in most individuals.

Lipodystrophy of the axillary folds and infrascapular area can produce a bulge above and below the brassiere, which patients regard as unsightly. Also, excess fat in the axillary folds area may cause chafing and an uncomfortable fit of clothing. Liposculpture to this area may improve appearance and comfort for appropriately selected patients.

The so-called dowager's hump is a fibrofatty mass of tissue that overlies the lower cervical or upper thoracic vertebrae. It varies in size from 10 to 25 cm in diameter and has various depths depending on the individual. This area, in addition to producing a cosmetic deformity, also may limit the range of motion in a person's neck. The results of this surgery can be very gratifying for the surgeon and the patient.

▷ Preoperative Evaluation

Examination should be performed with the patient in the standing position and the arm held extended with a 90-degree bend at the elbow, in order to properly evaluate the amount of excess adipose tissue and the elasticity of the adjacent skin. I have been able to perform liposculpture even on arms that are clinically quite large. The absolute size of the arms is less important than other factors. The important considerations are:

- ▶ The patient is of normal weight, or mildly to moderately overweight, in total body composition.
- ▶ The patient's forearms are not excessively obese.
- ▶ The patient has adequate skin elasticity.
- ▶ The patient is willing to pursue a regular regimen of simple exercise afterward to help contract the lax skin.
- ▶ The patient has realistic expectations of what can be achieved with the surgery.

As in all body liposculpture, a patient who has lost a large amount of weight rapidly is not considered a good candidate for this procedure. Patients with a recent absolute weight loss of more than 100 pounds may not be suitable candidates for liposculpture of the arms.

As with any liposculpture procedure, the patient must be carefully counseled as to the possibility of contour irregularities, persistent redundancy of the skin, and wrinkling of the skin.

▷ Surgical Procedure

Marking

With the patient standing, arm extended and bent upward 90 degrees at the elbow, the areas of excess adiposity are marked with a gentian violet marking pen (Fig. 15-1). The boundaries of the suction lines should be delineated by the me-

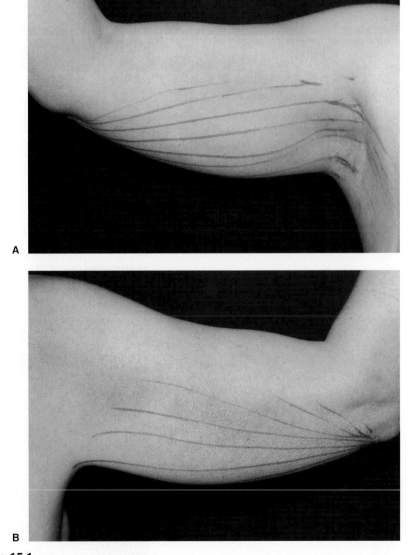

Figure 15-1

A,B: Preoperative markings for liposculpture surgery of the arms. Note single incision site above the elbow.

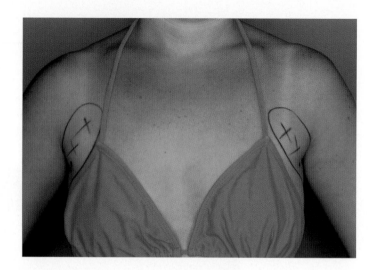

Figure 15-2

Preoperative markings for liposculpture surgery of the anterior axillary folds.

dial and lateral edges of the biceps muscle, so that the entire area below the muscle extending around the entire posterior aspect of the arm is included in the areas to be treated by liposculpture.

The anterior and posterior axillary folds can be treated in conjunction with the arms. Again, it is important to mark these areas with the patient in a standing position (Fig.15-2 to 15-4). One should carefully delineate the anterior axillary fold and its point of transition from the lateral breast.

If the infrascapular fat pad is to be treated, it should be marked at the same time, outlining its shape, which is usually at a 45-degree angle running parallel to the posterior flank (Fig. 15-4).

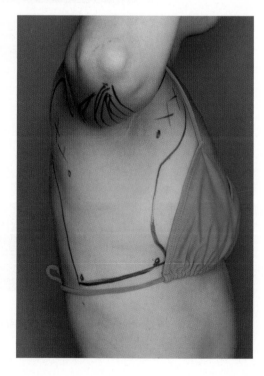

Figure 15-3

Preoperative markings for liposculpture surgery of the arms, anterior axillary folds, and posterior axillary folds.

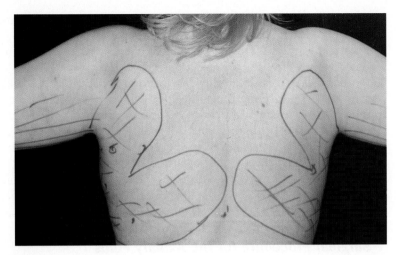

Figure 15-4
Preoperative markings for liposculpture surgery of the arms, posterior axillary folds, and infrascapular area.

If the dowager's hump is to be treated, the margins of the fatty protuberance are marked outlining its shape.

After marking, the area is infused in the usual fashion with tumescent solution containing 0.1% lidocaine.

Surgical Procedure for the Arms

The patient is placed in the prone position, with the arm extended laterally and held by a surgical assistant, with the forearm hanging in a downward position, forming a 90-degree angle with the arm. Having an assistant support the arm makes it easy to rotate the arm along the axis to be suctioned, and the surgeon can concentrate on sculpting the arm.

A single 2-mm incision is made in the midline of the posterior aspect of the arm just above the elbow. This is generally the only incision necessary for suctioning the upper arm.

In performing the surgery, it is important to utilize the appropriate size cannula and to suction at several different levels. Also, careful feathering on the lateral aspect of the area near the borders of the biceps muscle is very important. Nerve fibers must be carefully respected during the surgery, especially the radial and other nerves near the elbow and the abundance of nerve fibers in the axilla.

To begin the procedure, I use 12-gauge Klein spatula-type cannulas. I begin with a 4-inch cannula to treat the area immediately adjacent to the incision site. Then I extend to the 6-inch, 10-inch, and 12-inch cannulas, if needed, to reach from the incision site all the way toward the axilla. One should avoid entering the axilla itself because of the major arteries, veins, and nerves that are located there. This establishes the first level of suctioning for the arm, and it is midplane in depth.

Next, I use a Cook cannula, 3 mm in diameter, to approach the deeper plane proximate to the underlying fascia of the triceps muscle. After carefully traversing the area to ensure uniformity, I increase the diameter to a 3.5-mm Cook cannula, depending on the amount of excess adipose tissue, and again suction deep over the triceps muscle. This ensures removing the maximal amount of deep adipose tissue without causing any surface irregularities.

Following this, I carefully smooth the areas with a 12-inch 10-gauge Klein cannula to remove the remainder of the adipose tissue closest to the underlying musculature. Finally, I suction at a more superficial plane with 12-gauge Klein cannulas, again beginning with a 4 inch length and increasing in gradual increments to the 6-, 10-, and 12-inch cannulas to produce smooth results.

Periodically, the assistant rotates the arm upward with the posterior aspect of the arm facing downward and flexes the arm in a tightened biceps muscle position, so that I can observe the degree of contouring that has been achieved.

Surgical Procedure for the Axillary Folds

I utilize four 2-mm incisions: anteriorly at the mammary-axillary fold crease and at the inframammary crease, and posteriorly at the mid-post-axillary line and at the lower posterior axillary fold. While sculpting, one must be careful to respect the abundance of nerve fibers in this area.

Suctioning in this area is usually achieved satisfactorily with 12- and 14-gauge Klein spatula cannulas, 4 and 6 inches in length. Because of the soft nature of the axillary fold fat, especially anteriorly, it is best to avoid open-ended cannulas, which may easily oversuction the area or produce grooves.

The amount of fat removed from this region is small. However, the impact on the overall contouring procedure is significant, and the area should be treated when indication exists.

Surgical Procedure for the Infrascapular Fat Pad

The infrascapular fat pad is best suctioned through incisions in the superior post-axillary line, the lower post-axillary fold incision previously mentioned, and the midline of the back. Using these three incisions, one can crisscross the fold adequately and achieve good surgical results. (See Chapter 10 for a description of this procedure.)

Surgical Procedure for the Dowager's Hump

The area is infiltrated with standard tumescent solution. I generally use the formulation with a 0.1% concentration of lidocaine. The incisions are made at 3 o'clock, 6 o'clock, and 9 o'clock. This placement allows adequate treatment of the area with good crisscrossing and also provides an inferior drainage site.

Because the area is very dense and fibrous, small cannulas will generally be most advantageous in breaking up this fibrofatty tissue and achieving a higher degree of aspiration than is generally possible with the larger cannulas. Therefore, I generally begin the surgery with 4- to 6-inch 14-gauge Klein cannulas and 14-gauge Capistrano cannulas, followed by 12-gauge Klein and Capistrano cannulas. Then I utilize a 3-mm Pinto cannula to remove the thicker portions of the dowager fat pad. A final sculpting and blending is achieved with a 12-gauge Klein cannula.

This fibrofatty area may also be quite vascular in some individuals. Therefore, a good compression type of dressing should be applied postoperatively. I generally use 4 × 4 dressings pulled tightly over the area with stretch foam tape (3M).

▷ Postoperative Considerations

After completion of the sculpting of the arm, excess tumescent fluid is carefully expressed from the tissues to decrease the amount of drainage that the patient will experience postoperatively. As with all my liposculpture procedures, the incisions are left open to close spontaneously, which promotes good drainage. Absorbent dressings are placed over the incision sites, and a stocking-net type of compression dressing is placed over the entire upper arm (Fig. 15-5). If the axillary folds and infrascapular area have been treated, a compression vest garment is also utilized (see Figs. 10-4 and 16-2).

Patients should rest for the remainder of that day, making sure to maintain good hydration. They should keep their arms elevated as much as possible, especially during the first 24 hours.

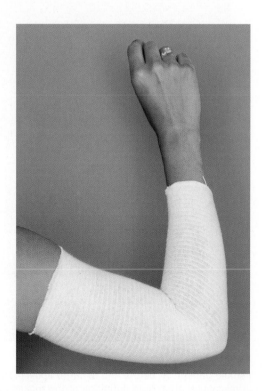

Figure 15-5
Patient wearing compressing dressing following liposculpture surgery of the arm.

The day after surgery they should take a shower and put on fresh absorbent dressings and a clean surgical garment. Patients may shower as often as they like during the postoperative period, but they should avoid water immersion, such as a swimming pool, hot tub, or bath, until all the incision sites have closed.

Patients are allowed to resume normal activities immediately. Triceps exercises twice a day are to be resumed 24 hours after surgery, using 3- to 5-pound weights, depending on the patient's age and strength. The importance of postoperative exercise on a twice-daily basis cannot be overstated.

Rarely, a patient will have temporary localized swelling above the elbow or in the axillary folds. If this occurs it can be treated by external ultrasound therapy and intralesional triamcinolone acetonide (Kenalog), 2.0 mg/mL, which generally causes it to resolve quickly.

The dowager's hump area tends to be very fibrous. In some cases it may be advantageous to treat it with Kenalog, 5 mg/mL or 10 mg/mL, and external ultrasound to reduce swelling.

In general, liposculpture of the posterior arm is user-friendly for the surgeon. If the basic guidelines described are followed and the surgeon suctions in the correct plane and in a uniform fashion across the extent of the arm, the possible complications of irregularities, depressions, and waviness can be avoided. In my practice, these problems are almost never seen. Patient satisfaction is usually high and recovery is very rapid.

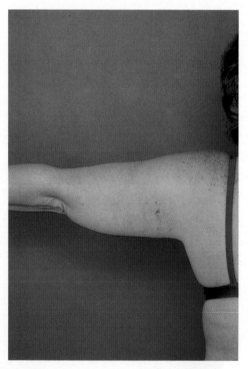 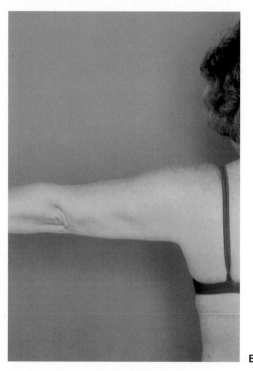

A   B

Figure 15-6

Female patient (**A**) before and (**B**) after liposculpture surgery of the arms, axillary folds, and infrascapular area. Note definition of the triceps muscle.

▷ Results

Following liposculpture surgery to the upper arm, the majority of patients notice a reduction of flabbiness and volume of the arm, with a smoother contour of the arm and better visual definition of the underlying triceps musculature (Fig. 15-6 to 15-8). Following liposculpture of the axillary folds and infrascapular areas, many patients report increased comfort, with less chafing in axillary areas and a reduced volume of the axillary folds and back. Patients have a more pleasing cosmetic appearance, with a reduction of fullness and bulging above and below the brassiere.

Liposculpture reduces the dowager's hump deformity and helps to restore a more normal contour to the neck and back, with increased mobility of the neck in many patients (Fig. 15-9).

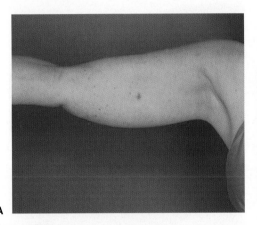 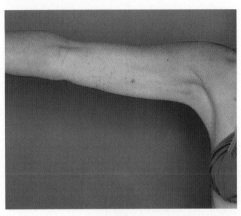

A   B

Figure 15-7
Female patient (**A**) before and (**B**) after liposculpture surgery of the arms. Note excellent tightening of the skin.

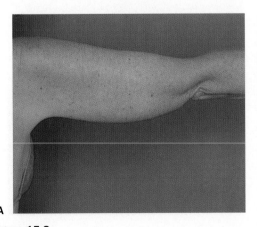 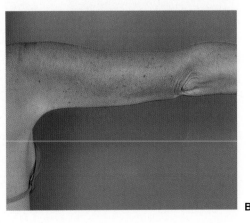

A   B

Figure 15-8
Female patient (**A**) before and (**B**) after liposculpture surgery of the arms. Note excellent tightening of the skin and definition of the triceps muscle.

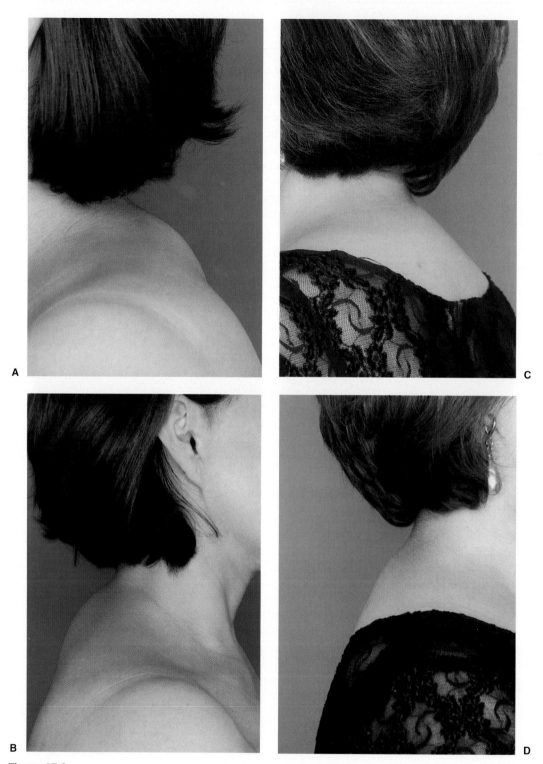

Figure 15-9

Female patient (**A,B**) before and (**C,D**) after liposculpture surgery of the so-called dowager's hump.

CHAPTER 16

LIPOSCULPTURE OF THE MALE BREASTS

Preoperative Evaluation ▶ *Surgical Procedure* ▶
Postoperative Considerations ▶ *Results*

Liposculpture of the breasts is currently limited primarily to the treatment of pseudogynecomastia in the adult male. I do not attempt to treat true gynecomastia, in which there is a proliferation of strictly glandular tissue. Female breast reduction using liposculpture is not discussed here, although several individuals are currently pursuing development of this technique. Any asymmetrical changes in breast size, in men or women, should be evaluated by good physical examination, appropriate biopsy, and open removal of glandular tissue when necessary.

The discussion in this chapter applies only to liposculpture for normal men who show a bilateral increase in size of the breasts, where the increase in size is primarily due to fatty tissue.

▷ Preoperative Evaluation

Most men with pseudogynecomastia display not only a physical and cosmetic disability, but also a large amount of psychological overlay. Many will not wear tight-fitting T-shirts or go to the beach because of embarrassment over this condition. Proper physical examination, discussion of the condition with the patient, and counseling are extremely important components of this surgery.

Pseudogynecomastia is common in 13- to 17-year-old boys, being reported as high as 38%. In this age group, it normally needs no evaluation or treatment and will resolve with time. Prepubertal gynecomastia is unusual and should be evaluated. Middle age or later gynecomastia is most susceptible to treatment by liposculpture. It is usually related to weight gain and/or decreased testicular function. One also must take a careful drug history in these patients.

In evaluating the patient, it is important to assess the patient's expectations and to discuss the surgical results that can realistically be achieved. If the breasts have a ptotic appearance, with the axis of the nipple pointing downward, the surgeon should be careful about accepting these patients for surgery. This ptotic effect will usually persist after surgery, so that the patient may not be fully satisfied with his results.

The patient must understand that the breast tissue itself, underlying the nipple and areola, will persist following the surgery. The relative proportion of glandular tissue to fatty tissue in the breast must be determined. The patient should be advised that open excision of glandular tissue might be necessary in selected cases.

It is very important to consider not only the breast area itself, but also the adjacent axillary folds that make up this cosmetic unit. Both the anterior and posterior axillary folds should be included in the sculpting, so that a pleasing contour of the breast, axillary region, and posterior axillary fold will be achieved in a true three-dimensional manner.

The highest patient satisfaction appears to be found when the abdomen is also treated at the same time, to achieve overall contouring of the entire area. (See Chapter 10 for a discussion of this procedure.)

▷ Surgical Procedure

One should carefully mark the areas of actual glandular tissue, the surrounding areas of lipodystrophy, and the region extending into the axilla. Marking is done with a gentian violet pen, with the patient in a sitting or standing position (Fig. 16-1).

I generally utilize the following four incisions: in the midline at approximately the 4 o'clock position; laterally at the 7 and 10 o'clock positions (these incisions also allow access to the axillary fold); and posteriorly in the posterior axillary line at approximately the level of the nipple.

I prefer tumescent solution containing 0.1% lidocaine for this region. As in all areas, it is a good idea to reinfiltrate with tumescent solution approximately halfway through the procedure. This expands the working space to achieve good yield, and also reinforces the vasoconstriction effect.

The chest area is always very fibrofatty and can be extremely dense in some individuals. Therefore, one generally needs to utilize more aggressive cannulas to achieve good contouring of the area. Small cannulas make the procedure easier for the surgeon. I begin with a 4-inch 14-gauge Klein spatula cannula to facilitate the breakup of the fibrofatty tissue, followed by a 6-inch 14-gauge Klein spatula cannula. To additionally loosen the fibrofatty tissue and begin extracting fatty material, I next use a 4- to 6-inch 14-gauge Capistrano cannula, followed by a 12-gauge Capistrano cannula. Finally, I use a 3-mm Pinto cannula, 15 cm in length, which is a more aggressive type of cannula and provides a good yield of aspirate. Care must be taken to crisscross the areas and to sculpt uniformly in all directions. The most concentrated effort will be needed in the periareolar region, where the fibrofatty tissue is much denser.

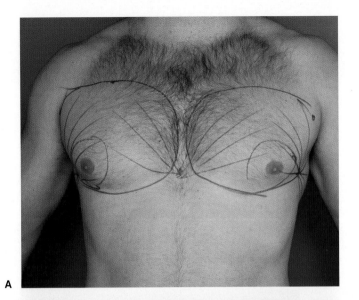

A

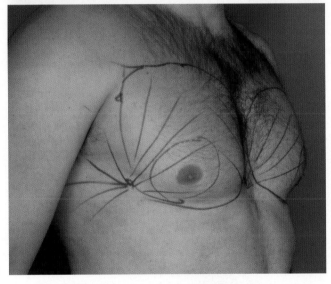

B

Figure 16-1
A,B: Preoperative markings for liposculpture surgery of the male breasts.

When suctioning in the other direction to treat the axillary fold, one must keep in mind that this tissue tends to be much softer and is easily removed, so that suctioning here should be less aggressive. Men tend to have smaller posterior axillary folds than women. Therefore, usually only one additional incision needs to be made in that area.

It is important to leave the inframammary crease region intact, because it provides support for the breast. When concurrent suctioning is being done on the abdomen, care should be taken not to penetrate the inframammary crease during the suctioning procedure.

In this region, the surgeon uses tactile and visual senses to achieve the final result. The incisions are not sutured, so that good drainage will occur.

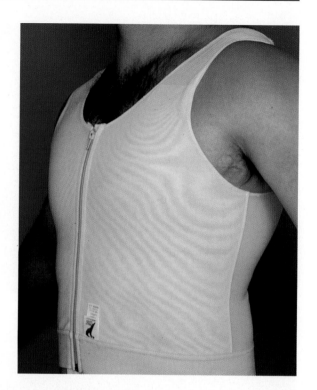

Figure 16-2

Male patient wearing surgical vest following liposculpture surgery of the breasts.

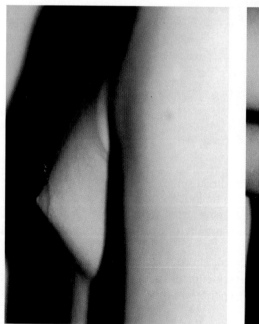

A

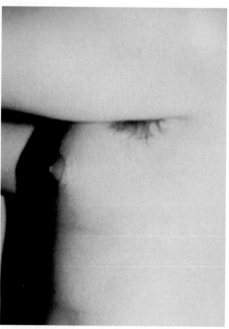

B

Figure 16-3

Male patient (**A**) before and (**B**) after liposculpture surgery of breasts.

▷ Postoperative Considerations

The chest area, being fibrofatty and vascular, requires good compression. A vest type surgical garment is useful for this purpose (Fig. 16-2). Absorbent pads are placed under the garment because of the drainage of tumescent fluid that will occur after surgery.

For the remainder of that day, patients should rest and maintain good hydration. In the morning, they should take a shower and then put on a clean surgical vest and dry absorbent pads. Patients may shower as often as they wish, but should avoid water immersion until all the incision sites have closed.

Patients are ambulatory immediately and are allowed to resume light exercise during the next several days. Postoperative exercises, especially those that work the chest muscle and build up the pectoral musculature, are recommended. They help the male patient to regain and maintain a good muscular physique.

▷ Results

Postoperatively the pseudogynecomastia is reduced and the chest has a more normal male contour (Fig. 16-3).

CHAPTER 17

BLEPHAROPLASTY

Surgical Use of the Pulsed CO$_2$ Laser ▶
Preoperative Evaluation ▶ *Preoperative Marking*
▶ *Operative Procedure* ▶ *Surgical Procedure* ▶
Postoperative Considerations ▶ *Results*

Patients who request liposculpture often exhibit a need for additional cosmetic procedures as well to gain the maximum improvement in appearance. In particular, patients who are undergoing the Cook Weekend Alternative to the Facelift™ (see Chapter 9) may benefit from eyelid rejuvenation. The main procedures I utilize in conjunction with the Cook Weekend Alternative to the Facelift™ are laser blepharoplasty and laser skin resurfacing, which may be combined with various forms of chemical peels. These procedures can maximize the ultimate result, clinically and on a structural basis, so that the eyes match the newly youthful appearance of the face, and the entire face, neck, and chest are rejuvenated due to the laying down of new collagen and reorganization of the elastic fibers in the skin.

I will describe my technique for laser blepharoplasty in this chapter. Techniques described apply to the "Western" eyelid. Specialized techniques exist for treating the Asian eyelid, and other texts should be consulted for these techniques. (See Chapter 18 for a discussion of skin resurfacing in combination with liposculpture procedures.)

▷ Surgical Use of the Pulsed CO$_2$ Laser

Advanced technology with the development of pulsed lasers, specifically the Coherent UltraPulse 5000 laser (see Appendix), which I utilize in my practice, allowed refinement of the blepharoplasty procedure so that patients have a much shortened recovery time, minimal bruising, and superior clinical results. These pulsed lasers emit interrupted beams of light, which produce less thermal injury and allow the targeted tissues to cool between pulses. Pulsed lasers produce less heat, less char, less coagulation necrosis, and less injury to tissues than earlier un-pulsed surgical lasers. The same pulsed laser technology may be used for resurfac-ing the skin, as discussed in Chapter 18.

The pulsed CO_2 laser has several advantages over traditional metal scalpel techniques in skin surgery. These advantages include: very precise ablation of tis-sue, less bleeding, less bruising, less postoperative discomfort, and a more rapid recovery and return to normal activity.

The small 0.2-mm laser spot size allows precise cutting and an unobstructed view during the making of the surgical incision. Also, it is felt that this laser is gen-tler to the tissues, with minimal thermal injury and no crush injury.

The decreased bleeding is an important advantage of the pulsed CO_2 lasers compared to traditional techniques. The laser produces an essentially bloodless field and seals small blood vessels of less than 0.5 mm in diameter. This gives the surgeon better visibility during the operation and lowers the postoperative risk of hemorrhage and ecchymosis.

The laser also seals small lymphatic vessels, which is felt to decrease postoper-ative swelling. This, in turn, decreases postoperative discomfort for the patient and allows for faster recovery.

Patients seem to note less discomfort and to require little postoperative pain medication. This decreased pain is felt to be due to sealing of the nerve endings by the laser. It has been noted histologically that cut nerve endings are sealed in the areas treated by the laser.

There are some disadvantages to use of the pulsed CO_2 laser. One is the ex-pense of the equipment. Others are the technical difficulties and the extended learning curve required for using this type of laser. There are serious safety issues associated with these lasers, so that the surgeon must carefully follow the impor-tant guidelines for electrical, fire, respiratory, and eye protection.

▷ Preoperative Evaluation

Indications for CO_2 pulsed laser cosmetic blepharoplasty include: excessive skin of the upper eyelids (dermatochalasis), indistinct or obscure supratarsal fold, protru-sions of fat in the upper and lower eyelids, and resectable xanthelasma. Patients will often present with nonspecific complaints such as "tired looking" eyes, baggy eyelids, and a desire to look younger. They may wish to have wrinkling in the peri-orbital and facial areas corrected, or dark circles under the eyes minimized.

It is important to discuss realistic expectations. Demonstrate to the patient the anticipated result by pulling up the skin of the upper eyelids with a cotton-tipped swab. The anticipated recovery time from the procedure should also be discussed.

During the examination, press gently on the globe to note any fatty protru-sion in the lower eyelids. Also, it is important to note at this time any deformities that may be present, especially any lower eyelid laxity. It is helpful to test eyelid and orbicularis tone with an eyelid retraction maneuver. The eyelid is pulled away from the globe and allowed to snap back, to determine if the eyelid has enough elasticity to withstand a surgical procedure. If the snapback is poor, the patient may need to be evaluated for a lower eyelid tightening procedure.

Some of the contraindications to the CO_2 laser cosmetic blepharoplasty include: uncontrolled hypertension, active Grave's disease, proptosis greater than 3 mm, unstable or uncontrolled glaucoma, serious retinal disease, severe dry-eye syndrome (keratitis sica), and acute blepharitis. Relative contraindications would include: shallow orbit, deep-set eyes, asymmetry, ptosis, proptosis, and hypotonia of the lower eyelid. Patients should understand that the procedure will not remove cheek pads (known as malar fat pads).

The blepharoplasty procedure is commonly done in combination with the Cook Weekend Alternative to the Facelift™ (see Chapter 9). The same presurgical regimen is prescribed, with prophylactic antibiotics and prophylactic antiviral medications.

▷ Preoperative Marking

I use a gentian violet pen to mark the eyelids, with the patient sitting in the upright position with the eyes gently closed. In marking the lower eyelid, close the eyes and gently press on the globe to protrude the fat pads (Fig. 17-1). Outline the protrusion on the eyelid, especially noting the lateral fat pad, which can be the most difficult to remove.

In the upper eyelid, I look for the natural crease of the supratarsal fold, which is usually 6 to 8 mm above the eyelid margin (Fig. 17-2). Use tenotomy forceps to estimate excess skin (Fig. 17-3). Plan to leave an average of 10 to 12 mm of skin between the upper incision and the inferior hairs of the eyebrow. Follow the

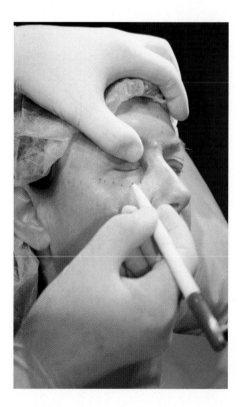

Figure 17-1
Preoperative markings of the lower eyelid fat pad.

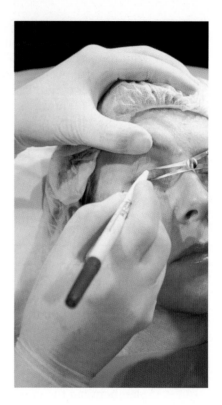

Figure 17-2
Preoperative markings of the supratarsal fold, which is measured from the upper eyelid margin.

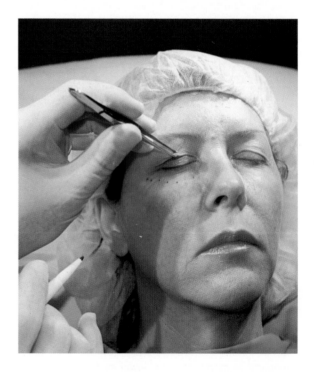

Figure 17-3
Use of tenotomy forceps to estimate excess skin of the upper eyelid.

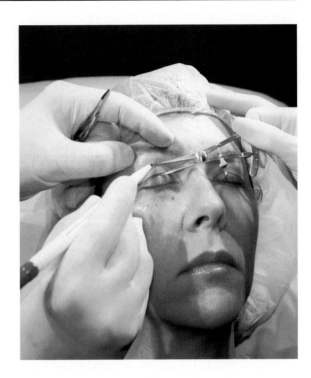

Figure 17-4
Preoperative markings showing incision on
the upper eyelid.

natural curve of the tarsal plate. The medial margin of the incision should be
planned to be even with the lacrimal punctum. The lateral extension of the excision is best kept within the confines of the orbit (Fig. 17-4).

▷ Surgical Procedure

The surgeon must have detailed knowledge of the eye and eyelid anatomy. Operative errors in these regions are unforgiving. Accurate placement of the supratarsal
fold is critical. Also, one must be careful not to disrupt the pretarsal orbicularis
muscle, which is the supporting sling for the tarsal plate.

Laser safety is especially important during blepharoplasty. Metal protective
shields must be used for the cornea and globe. Wet towels should be placed
around the field, covering the face and nonoperative areas. No volatile skin prepa-
rations or anesthetics should be used and no oxygen should be flowing. All plastic tubes should be covered. Smoke should be evacuated during the procedure.
Special laser masks should be available for use by the surgical staff. The surgeon
and all personnel in the operating room should also have protective eyewear in
place during the procedure.

A constant smooth sweeping arc should always be utilized for the laser beam.
Any hesitation or tremor gives a jagged line. A long pause in any area may burn
the tissues.

I perform blepharoplasty immediately after the Cook Weekend Alternative to
the Facelift™. Just before suturing the submental incision to complete that procedure, I infiltrate the lower eyelids with 2% xylocaine with 1:100,000

epinephrine (see subsequent text). This allows adequate time for anesthesia and vasoconstriction to be achieved, so that as soon as the submental wound is closed, I can begin the blepharoplasty procedure. I always do the lower eyelids first and then the upper eyelids, infiltrating the next eyelid just before I begin treatment of the preceding area.

Surgical Procedure for the Lower Eyelids

I prefer to approach the lower eyelid via the conjunctiva, rather than operating through the skin. Transconjunctival lower eyelid CO_2 laser blepharoplasty has many advantages. Among these are that the orbital septum is not violated; there is no skin excision, therefore, no scar; there is less retraction of the eyelid; the procedure itself is quicker and easier, with few complications; and it is less likely to change the shape of the lower eyelid.

There are risks associated with transconjunctival lower eyelid blepharoplasty that must be avoided. These include the danger of injury to the inferior oblique muscle and the possibility of lasing through the eyelid skin.

The lower eyelid anesthesia is directed through the conjunctival surface. First a topical anesthetic ophthalmic solution such as proparacaine (Ophthane) is applied. Then, approximately 5 to 7 mm down from the ciliary margin, a single penetration is made through the conjunctival surface. One should extend the 1-inch 30-gauge needle to the orbital rim, back off slightly, and then inject approximately 2 mL of the 2% xylocaine/1:100,000 epinephrine mixture. Care should be taken to avoid the arcade of vessels on the conjunctival surface. Immediately after injection, place firm pressure on the area for approximately 5 minutes to dissipate the solution, as well as to control bleeding. It is very important to achieve pressure hemostasis at this time. Injection hematomas can be a very serious consequence and certainly should be avoided if possible.

Begin the procedure by retracting the lower eyelid anteriorly with a Ball retractor. Insert the Jaeger bone plate into the inferior fornix, with pressure on the plate to cause bulging of the fat outwardly and anteriorly.

Utilizing the Coherent UltraPulse 5000 laser in its 7-W continuous-wave, slightly defocused setting, make the conjunctival incision approximately 4 to 5 mm below the eyelid margin in the first pass (Fig. 17-5). The second pass encompasses the capsulopalpebral fascia and eyelid retractors. The third pass opens the compartment so that the fat bulges out.

The middle pad is removed first. Grab it gently with forceps and tease it free. Inject it with 2% xylocaine with 1:100,000 epinephrine. Place a wet cotton-tip applicator or Byron pineapple metal surface behind it and remove the fat with the laser on the 7-W continuous-wave setting.

The lateral fat pad is removed next. Extend the incision laterally. Press on the skin of the lateral orbit to visualize the fat bulge. Inject it with 2% xylocaine with 1:100,000 epinephrine. Place a wet cotton-tip applicator or Byron pineapple metal surface behind it and remove the fat.

Finally, remove the medial fat pad by extending the incision medially. The whitish fat will be visible. This area is more sensitive and contains many angular

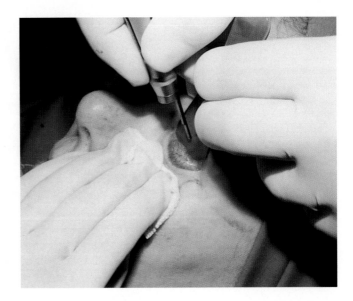

Figure 17-5
Operative procedure for transconjunctival lower lid blepharoplasty. Making the conjunctival incision.

vessels, which must be carefully cauterized with the Valley electrosurgical unit (see Appendix) to ensure good hemostasis. The medial fat pad is removed in the same manner as the middle fat pad.

There are some important techniques to keep in mind when performing transconjunctival lower eyelid blepharoplasty. Do not pull on the fat; treat only that fat which is easily grasped by the forceps. Use gentle pressure on the globe to make the fat bulge flush with the orbital rim. Be sure to check for redraping of the lower eyelid skin with gentle pressure on the globe.

It is not necessary to close the lower eyelid conjunctival incision. This area heals very rapidly and without problems. Sutures in this area should be avoided because they can produce irritation and, possibly, corneal abrasion.

Surgical Procedure for the Upper Eyelids

A 1-inch 30-gauge needle is used to inject the anesthetic. The injection is positioned as a single penetration type of stick in the midline of the upper eyelid. Approximately 2 mL of the 2% xylocaine/1:100,000 epinephrine mixture is injected into the marked area. As with the lower eyelids, pressure is immediately applied to the area for approximately 3 to 5 minutes. While the pressure is applied, the solution should be milked laterally and medially by a slow rocking motion over the injected bleb, so as to dissipate the solution into the eyelid. This technique avoids multiple penetrations, so it reduces the chance of injection hematoma and keeps bruising to a minimum.

For the initial skin incision, I utilize a 15-mJ, 4-W setting on the Coherent UltraPulse 5000 laser in pulse mode. The pass is completed in a fluid motion,

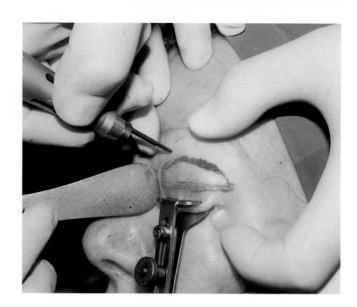

Figure 17-6

Operative procedure for upper lid blepharoplasty. Making the initial skin incision.

completely outlining the area to be excised. Then a 7-W continuous-wave setting is used for the skin and muscle excision (Fig. 17-6).

The skin and orbicularis muscle are removed as a unit, proceeding from lateral to medial. The medial canthal area should be protected from wave scatter with a Jaeger bone plate placed medially. A moistened cotton-tip applicator or Byron pineapple metal surface behind the flap of tissue will protect underlying tissues.

First, remove the middle fat pad (Fig. 17-7). After the septum has been exposed, it should be excised transversely over the bulging fat pad, putting gentle pressure on the globe to locate the fat pad. Extend the septal incision medially and laterally. Tease the middle fat pad free and inject it with 2% xylocaine with 1:100,000 epinephrine. Coagulate any large vessels over the surface with an elec-

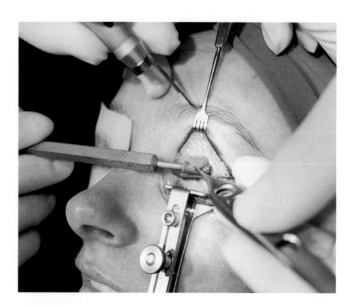

Figure 17-7

Operative procedure for upper lid blepharoplasty. Removing the middle fat pad.

trocautery unit such as the Valley electrosurgical unit. Then excise the middle fat pad with the laser on a continuous-wave defocused 7-W setting.

Next, remove the medial fat pad. This tends to be whitish fat and at times may be difficult to locate. The area is more sensitive and contains abundant angular vessels, which must be carefully electrocoagulated. Tease the medial fat pad free. Coagulate the vessels, and then remove the fat pad with the laser on continuous wave defocused mode. Check thoroughly at this point for good complete hemostasis.

There is no lateral fat pad in the upper eyelid. The lacrimal gland occupies this position.

Closure of the upper eyelid incision is accomplished utilizing 6-0 rapidly absorbing catgut interrupted sutures. Approximately 6 to 8 sutures are positioned. In the interspaces between them I utilize tissue glue, which additionally strengthens the incisions (Fig. 17-8). This method of closing allows the patient a fast recovery. The tissue glue and sutures will fall out in approximately 7 days.

Resurfacing

I have found that it is important to resurface the periorbital skin in the medial canthal area, even if more extensive resurfacing is not contemplated. For this I use the collimated handpiece of the Coherent UltraPulse laser, on the 300-mJ, 2-W setting, in one single pass over the medial canthus. It is very important that no wiping should be done after the laser pass. This resurfacing helps tighten the medial canthus skin without having to extend the excision into that area and allows for very quick healing of the area. It does not significantly extend the patient's recovery time. Sometimes, I will resurface the entire upper eyelid, or the upper and

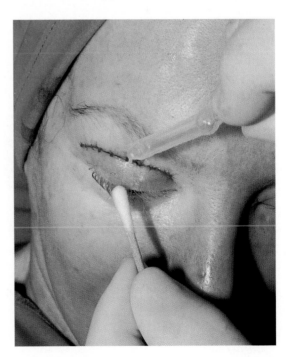

Figure 17-8

Operative procedure for upper lid blepharoplasty. Applying tissue glue to the upper eyelid incision site. Note the absence of ecchymosis on the upper and lower eyelids.

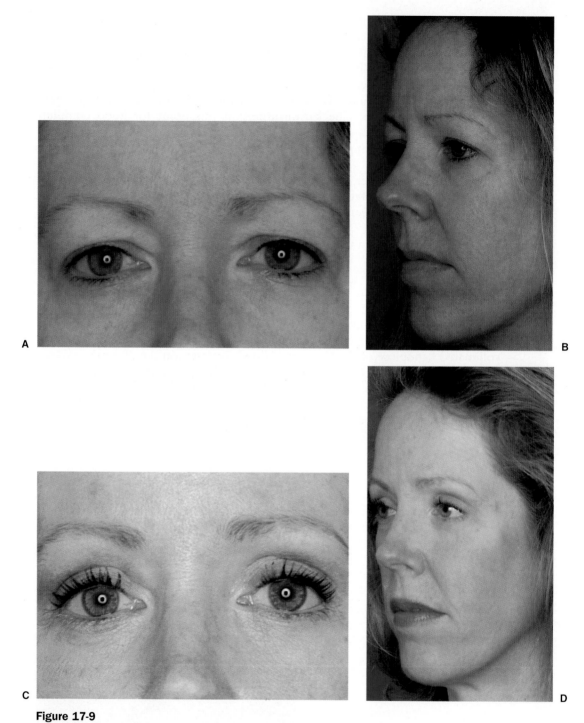

Figure 17-9

Female patient (**A,B**) before and (**C,D**) after blepharoplasty of the upper and lower eyelids without resurfacing.

lower eyelids, at the same time as the blepharoplasty procedure. (See Chapter 18 for details of complete periorbital laser resurfacing.)

▷ Postoperative Considerations

Postoperatively, patients are instructed to limit their activities for 2 days and to keep the head elevated 30 degrees while sleeping. They should use ice packs on the treated areas as much as possible during the remainder of the day of surgery, 15 minutes "on" and 15 minutes "off." Coughing should be avoided. Stress, lifting, and bending are to be avoided. Limiting activities immediately after eyelid surgery helps to speed recovery.

It is important to continue any antihypertensive medications to avoid high blood pressure. Antibiotics and antiviral medications should be continued. An artificial tears (Lacrilube) preparation may occasionally be used if the patient's eyes feel dry in the immediate postoperative period.

After 2 days patients may perform normal duties. However, they should still avoid excessive exercise or any activities that might elevate the blood pressure. Because the effects of pressurization and altitude can intensify swelling as well as possibly ecchymosis in some individuals in the immediate postoperative period, I recommend that patients not fly for at least 4 days after surgery. In my experience, if instructions are followed carefully, almost all patients experience little or no ecchymosis postoperatively.

If any hypertrophic healing of the upper eyelid incision develops, the area should be injected with intralesional triamcinolone acetonide (Kenalog), 2 to 5 mg/mL. This result is very uncommon in my experience and is easily treated.

In performing laser blepharoplasty, it is very important to follow safety guidelines. Reproducible results will be achieved with consistent surgical techniques.

▷ Results

Patients are generally very happy with the results of laser blepharoplasty (Figs. 17-9 to 17-15). When the Cook Alternative to the Facelift™ is combined with blepharoplasty, the overall cosmetic result is greatly enhanced. When blepharoplasty is combined with laser resurfacing of the eyelids, periorbital wrinkling is minimized and skin texture is improved. The eyelids have a more natural appearance postoperatively, with reduced drooping and "bagginess." Patients report that they have a less tired appearance and a brighter expression, and they feel that they look younger.

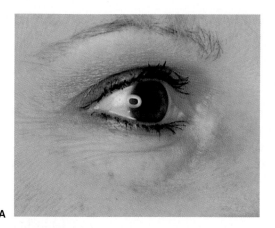
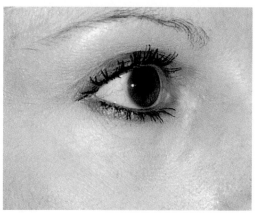

A   B

Figure 17-10

Patient (**A**) before and (**B**) after transconjunctival lower eyelid blepharoplasty without resurfacing.

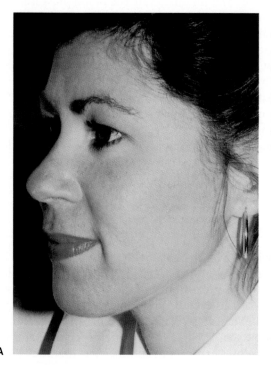
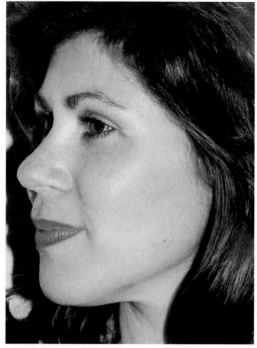

A   B

Figure 17-11

Patient (**A**) before and (**B**) after blepharoplasty of the upper and lower eyelids without resurfacing.

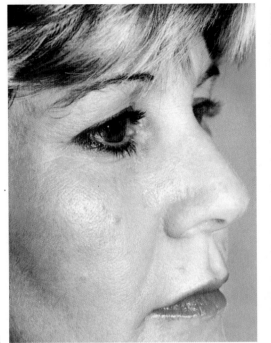
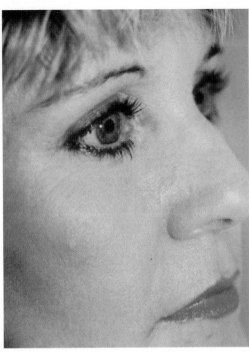

A   B

Figure 17-12
Patient (**A**) before and (**B**) after blepharoplasty of the upper eyelids without resurfacing.

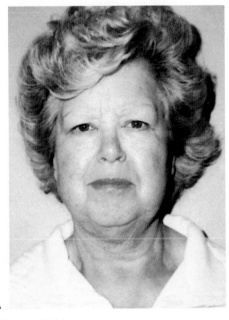
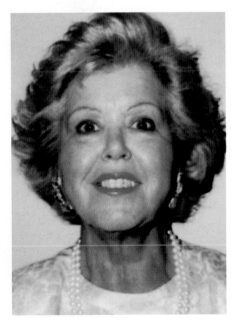

A   B

Figure 17-13
Patient (**A**) before and (**B**) after blepharoplasty of the upper eyelids combined with the Cook
Weekend Alternative to the Facelift™.

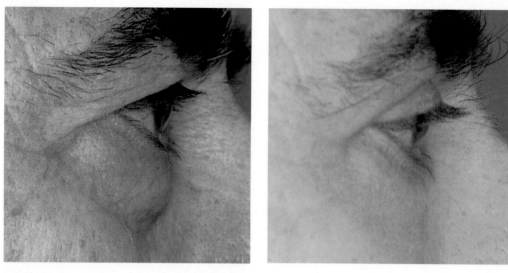

A   B

Figure 17-14

Patient (**A**) before and (**B**) after blepharoplasty of the upper eyelids and periocular laser resurfacing of the upper and lower eyelids.

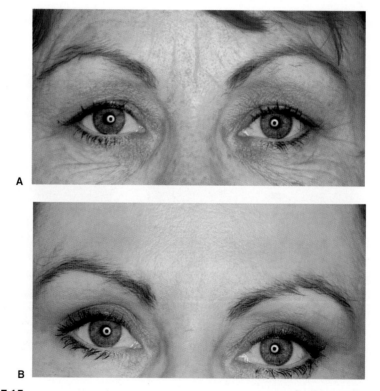

Figure 17-15

Patient (**A**) before and (**B**) after blepharoplasty of the upper eyelids and laser resurfacing of the entire face.

CHAPTER 18

SKIN RESURFACING AND BODY PEELS

Resurfacing the Nonfacial Skin ▶ *Preoperative Evaluation* ▶ *Procedures* ▶ *Postoperative Considerations* ▶ *Results*

In about 5% to 10% of patients undergoing the Cook Weekend Alternative to the Facelift™ procedure, we also resurface the face, neck, chest, and hands, either a few weeks before the surgery or a few days following the procedure. Patients seeking cosmetic surgery often show many epidermal and dermal lesions, such as irregular pigmentation, lentigines, keratoses, wrinkling, roughness, and other problems caused by sun damage and aging skin. For maximal improvement in their appearance, skin resurfacing with a laser or chemical peel in selected patients can greatly increase patient satisfaction. This treatment not only minimizes wrinkles, rough texture, and pigmented lesions, but it gives the skin a more vigorous and youthful quality, due to the formation of new collagen and reorganization of the elastic fibers in the skin.

▷ Resurfacing the Nonfacial Skin

Resurfacing treatments have traditionally been limited to the face, because standard techniques have not proven satisfactory for nonfacial skin. Superficial chemical peels of the nonfacial skin are too light to produce the desired results. Uncontrolled medium or deep peels of the nonfacial skin can give unpredictable results and may penetrate beyond the desired depth.

However, when just the face is resurfaced, the result can be a sharp line of demarcation between the treated skin of the face and the untreated skin of the neck and chest. This result gives an unnatural looking appearance and leaves the patient with a less than optimal result. For this reason, we have developed a method of "controlled" chemical peeling, which has proven to be safe and effective in peeling nonfacial skin. We call this technique the Cook Total Body Peel. (The term "total body peel" does not mean that we peel the entire body of every patient, but rather that the technique can be used on any part of the body.)

The Cook Total Body Peel can be performed on all areas of the body and on all skin types. This technique produces a peel ranging in depth from light to medium. It is entirely technique-dependent because the physician controls depth. We have used this technique for the past 7 years on over 2,000 patients with consistently good results on the neck, chest, hands, arms, legs, back, and indeed all areas of the body. The Cook Total Body Peel is particularly helpful in patients with freckled or actinically damaged necks, chests, and hands.

▷ Preoperative Evaluation

Patients must be examined carefully to determine which laser or peeling technique is indicated for their particular cosmetic concern, and also which peeling agent or laser technique would suit their lifestyle. At times, a combination of laser and chemical peels is used on various parts of the face for a more customized peel. We are always careful to respect cosmetic units, so that each area will blend smoothly with adjacent areas.

Factors that we consider in evaluating a patient include:

- ▶ Fitzpatrick skin type (1)
- ▶ Degree of actinic or age damage
- ▶ Prior cosmetic surgery
- ▶ General medical and physical condition of the patient
- ▶ Any history of hypertrophic healing, keloids, allergies, or acne
- ▶ Current medications, including isotretinoin (Accutane)
- ▶ Whether or not the patient uses foundation type cosmetics
- ▶ The degree of sun exposure that the patient currently experiences and will experience in the future
- ▶ The degree and extent of poikiloderma on the neck, and whether it extends onto the facial areas
- ▶ Whether the patient has realistic expectations

In evaluating prior cosmetic surgery, one must check for areas of previous cicatrix, ectropion, or scleral show. Also, it is important to obtain the history of any allergies, including "sensitive skin," so that the postoperative regimen can be adjusted appropriately. If the patient has a history of acne, the postoperative use of emollients should be less extensive and for a shorter period of time. For deeper laser peels, we require a medical clearance from a primary physician.

If the facial skin damage is severe, we recommend a facial peel using the Coherent Ultra-Pulse 5000 CO_2 laser or the Erbium:YAG laser. This resurfacing allows the improvement of wrinkles, actinic damage, and pigmentation, and reverses the loss of elasticity that may be noted in "aging" skin. Acne scars are also improved with this resurfacing technology. If the damage is only moderate, a facial peel using trichloroacetic acid (TCA) is recommended. Whenever a facial resurfacing is performed, either laser or chemical, we also treat the neck, chest, hands, and other indicated nonfacial areas using the Cook Total Body Peel technique.

Typically, male patients, because they do not wear makeup and have the most severe wrinkling around the eyelids, will receive a CO_2 laser peel to the periorbital area, with a TCA peel or Erbium:YAG peel to the remainder of the face. Patients with minimal periorbital wrinkling are given an Erbium:YAG or TCA peel to the entire face.

In most cases, we schedule the resurfacing treatment for either 3 to 4 weeks before the Cook Weekend Alternative to the Facelift™ procedure, or 3 to 5 days after it.

Before any skin resurfacing procedure, the patient is placed on prophylactic antibiotics and antiviral medication. We generally prescribe cefadroxil (Duricef), 500 mg b.i.d., and valacyclovir hydrochloride (Valtrex), 500 mg b.i.d., being careful to review the patient's allergic status with regard to both medications. If patients can tolerate tretinoin (Retin-A), they will benefit from preoperative application to the face. Alpha-hydroxy acids and hydroquinone may also be used. However, we prefer that patients not use high concentrations of alpha-hydroxy acids or tretinoin on nonfacial skin for 1 week prior to the procedure, as it increases the speed of penetration of the peeling substance.

▷ Procedures

Laser Peel

For a laser peel of the face, the areas to be treated are marked in the usual fashion (Figs. 18-1, 18-2). Patients are pretreated with intramuscular meperidine hydrochloride (Demerol) and midazolam (Versed). After nerve blocks, the face is infused with tumescent solution (Fig. 18-3). We use a solution containing (per 1,000 mL) a total of: 50 mL of 2% Xylocaine, 1 mL epinephrine (1:1000), 12.5 mEq of sodium bicarbonate, and 10 mg of triamcinolone acetonide (Kenalog). (See Chapter 5 for a discussion of the use of tumescent anesthesia.)

Either the Ultra-Pulse 5000 CO_2 laser or the Coherent Erbium:YAG laser is used for resurfacing the facial skin (Fig. 18-4). With the Ultra-Pulse 5000 laser we use the computer pattern generator (CPG) handpiece with a pattern setting of 3, scan size 5 to 9 mm, density 5 to 6, and energy 300 mJ, performing two to four laser passes. The transition area from the face to the neck is treated with a lower energy of 200 mJ and a lower density of 4, for better blending. The Coherent Erbium:YAG laser is used with a fluence of 5, CPG pattern 3, density 5, and two to five passes.

TCA Peel

In performing a TCA peel of the face, the patient is pretreated with intramuscular Demerol and Versed. No local anesthetic is used. The skin is cleansed with acetone, and a 40% TCA preparation is applied to the point of blanching. The skin is

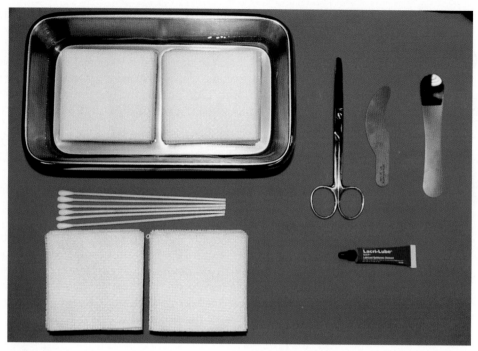

Figure 18-1

Instrument tray for laser peel: top, gauze sponges in sterile water, scissors, curved Jaeger plate, Jaeger bone plate; bottom, cotton-tip applicators, dry sponges, and Lacrilube.

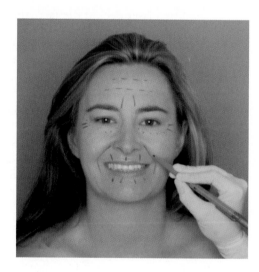

Figure 18-2

Preoperative markings for full face laser resurfacing.

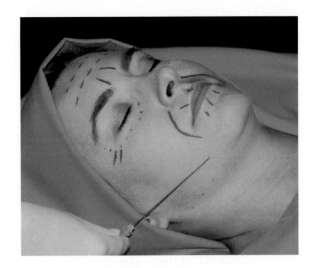

Figure 18-3

Infiltration of tumescent solution for full face laser resurfacing.

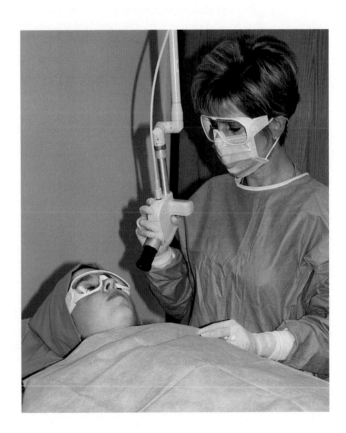

Figure 18-4

Laser peel of the face.

then neutralized with 10% sodium bicarbonate solution at the appropriate time, based on the degree of blanching desired.

Eyelid Peel

The extent of treatment of the eyelids depends on the degree of laxity of the lower eyelid margin. This may be determined by a snapback test (see Chapter 17). Also, the degree of wrinkling on the lower eyelid is a clue to the amount of eyelid laxity present: the less wrinkling there is, the more laxity is present. If the eyelid laxity is great, then one must carefully consider whether to do any resurfacing technique at all on the lower eyelid.

In patients who exhibit a poor snapback test and no lower eyelid wrinkling, we either do no peel at all or else do a light TCA peel. If there is moderate eyelid laxity and wrinkling on the lower eyelid, we may do one pass with the Ultra-Pulse 5000 CO_2 laser. If there is no eyelid laxity and the lower eyelid skin shows significant cosmetic problems, we perform two passes with the CO_2 laser. We use the CPG handpiece at a setting of 300 mJ. The first pass uses the settings: pattern 3, size 5, and density 5. The second pass is set at pattern 3, size 5, and density 3.

On the upper eyelid, we use the CO_2 laser with the CPG handpiece and pattern 3, size 5, density 6. We treat the entire eyelid down to the eyelashes on the first pass. If an upper eyelid blepharoplasty is being performed immediately after the resurfacing, the ellipse of skin that will be removed is not resurfaced. Then a second pass is given to the lateral one-half of the eyelid, from just under the eyebrow down to the supratarsal fold.

Cook Total Body Peel

This controlled chemical peel technique uses a combination of glycolic acid gel and TCA. Neutralization with sodium bicarbonate solution permits precise timing and limitation of the extent and depth of the peel.

No pretreatment with intramuscular or local anesthetic is needed. No sedation is required. The skin is cleansed with acetone. Then a 70% glycolic acid gel is applied with a folded 4 × 4 gauze, followed immediately by 40% TCA (Fig. 18-5). Several additional coats of TCA may be applied with a folded 4 × 4 gauze as needed until the desired depth is obtained. The skin must be carefully observed so that the physician can neutralize the peel at the desired depth with a copious amount of 10% sodium bicarbonate solution, applied at least five times and being careful to remove all glycolic acid gel from the skin.

The end point of each area is determined by the physician according to the patient's skin type, actinic damage, and "age damage." A typical end point is characterized by erythema with small scattered white speckles or an expression by the patient of a slight burning sensation (Fig. 18-6). In patients with darker skin types and less sun damage, the physician should limit the depth of the peel by neutralizing earlier. The upper neck should be peeled "deeper" than more distal areas of the neck and chest for better blending with the resurfaced face.

The artistry of the Cook Total Body Peel lies in the blending effect and consistency in depth of the peel on the various body areas. Careful attention to the

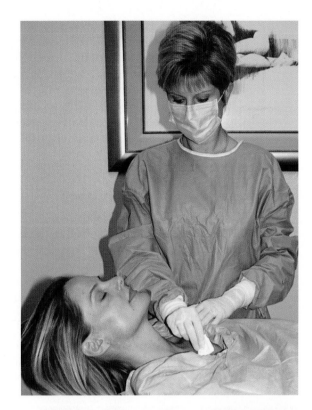

Figure 18-5

Solution being applied to the chest for a Cook Total Body Peel.

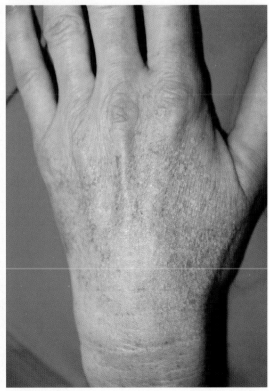

Figure 18-6

Cook Total Body Peel of the hand, showing end-point of speckled white on erythematous skin. Note that the lentigines and actinic keratoses have blanched more deeply.

color change (end point) is key to the cosmetic result. If certain skin areas require more time or more TCA to "speckle" to the same degree as neighboring skin, the physician can allow more time or apply more TCA before neutralization.

The result should be a lighter peel than a typical 40% TCA peel. This is in contrast to medium depth peels using TCA plus glycolic acid liquid. It is important to use glycolic acid gel for this technique, rather than liquid, because the gel acts as a partial barrier to the TCA penetration. Liquid glycolic acid does not act as a barrier and can result in complications by causing too deep a peel on the body.

▷ Postoperative Considerations

If possible, we like to have all patients use retinoic acid and hydroquinone in the postoperative period. Sun exposure should be strictly avoided for approximately 1 month following treatment.

Facial resurfacing patients are placed on emollients or a Flexzan type of dressing (Mylan Laboratories, Inc., Pittsburgh, PA), depending on the depth of the resurfacing. We prefer that patients not exercise extensively until reepithelialization.

Patients who have had a CO_2 laser peel are put on a standard laser peel postoperative regimen with Flexzan dressing (2). The skin will usually reepithelialize in 7 to 10 days, depending on the depth of the laser peel. The patient should not

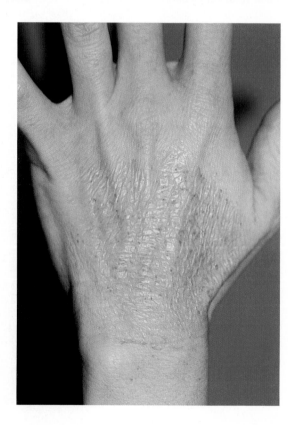

Figure 18-7

Cook Total Body Peel of the hand, approximately 1 week after the peel, showing the distal part of the hand already peeled and the proximal part of the hand in the process of peeling.

wear makeup until reepithelialization has occurred.

Patients who have had a TCA facial peel and Cook Total Body Peel are instructed to bathe several times a day and then reapply emollient. After a TCA peel, the skin will turn brown and peel between days 5 and 7. As soon as this process is completed, usually about day 7, the patient may return to work and other normal activities and may resume wearing makeup.

After a Cook Total Body Peel, the treated skin will peel in the form of flaking and scaling for 2 to 4 weeks postoperatively, depending on the area treated (Fig. 18-7). This is not usually a major cosmetic concern because the body areas can be covered with clothing. The Cook Total Body Peel can be repeated as often as every month, as soon as the flaking is complete.

The Cook Total Body Peel shows a significantly decreased incidence of postinflammatory pigmentation as compared to TCA alone. If postinflammatory pigmentation occurs, it resolves quickly with local hydroquinone treatment. We have not seen any scarring or other major complications with these techniques.

▷ Results

When a laser or chemical peel of the face is combined with a Cook Total Body Peel of the neck, there is excellent blending of the face and neck skin (Figs. 18-8 to 18-

(text continues on page 186)

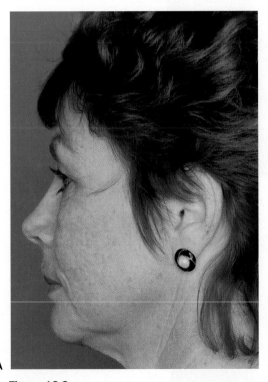 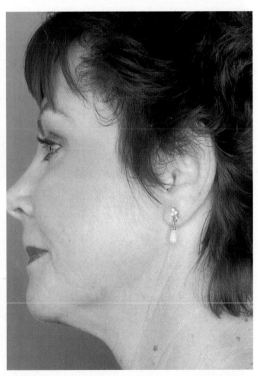

A   B

Figure 18-8
Patient (**A**) before and (**B**) after blending of full face laser peel with Cook Total Body Peel of the neck.

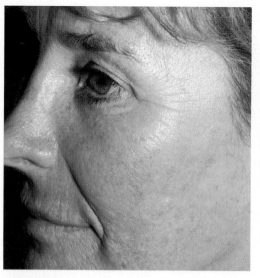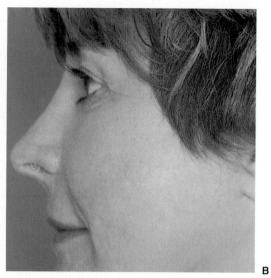

Figure 18-9

Patient (**A**) before and (**B**) after blending of full face laser peel with Cook Total Body Peel of the neck.

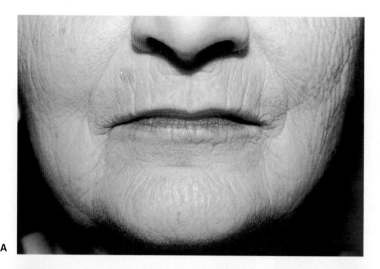

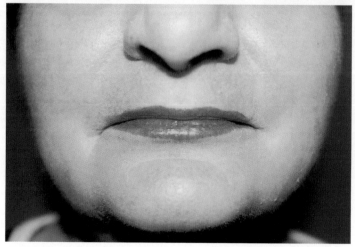

Figure 18-10

Patient (**A**) before and (**B**) after full face laser peel.

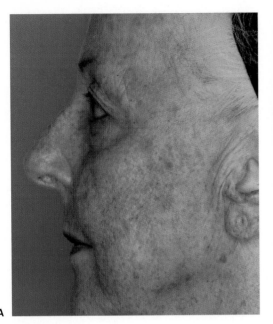
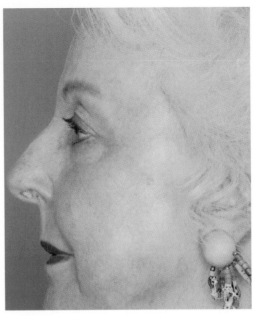

A

B

Figure 18-11

Patient (**A**) before and (**B**) after blending of full face laser peel with Cook Total Body Peel of the neck.

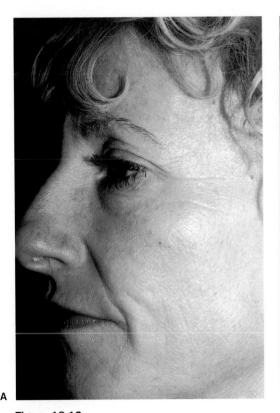
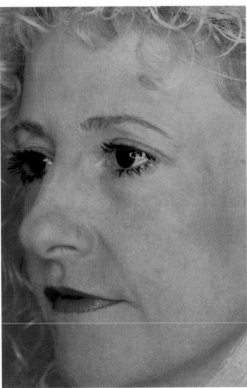

A

B

Figure 18-12

Patient (**A**) before and (**B**) after full face laser peel. Note diminished lines and tightened skin.

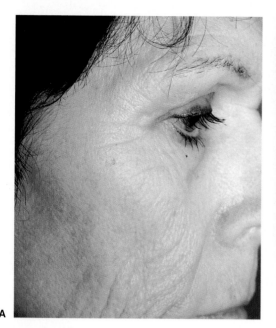 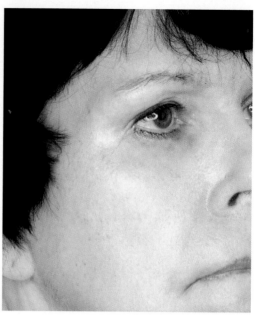

A
B

Figure 18-13

Patient (**A**) before and (**B**) after full face laser peel. Note dramatically tightened skin and reduced wrinkles.

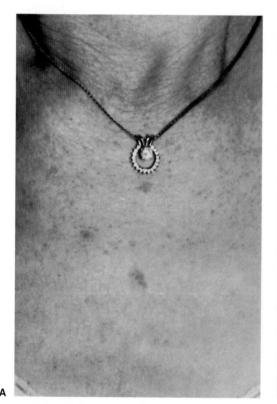 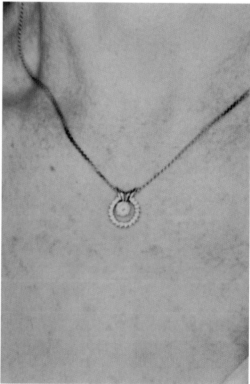

A
B

Figure 18-14

Patient (**A**) before and (**B**) after Cook Total Body Peel of neck and chest. One peel. Note improved texture of neck and chest skin.

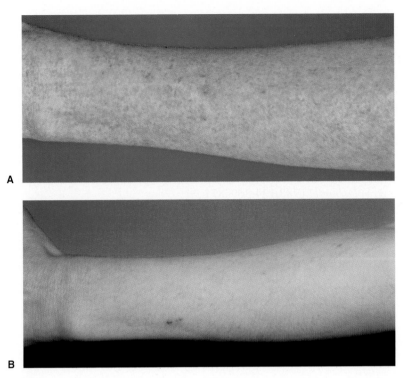

Figure 18-15

Patient (**A**) before and (**B**) after Cook Total Body Peel of the arms. One peel. (Note: The patient was accidentally scratched by a cat subsequent to the peel.)

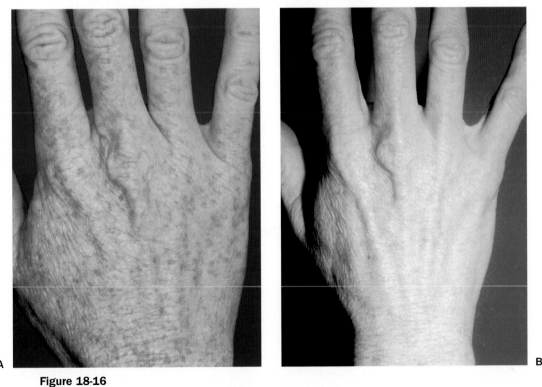

Figure 18-16

Patient (**A**) before and (**B**) after Cook Total Body Peel of the hands. One peel. Note lightening of the freckling on the hand and fingers.

185

13). The Cook Total Body Peel can be applied to the neck and chest (Fig. 18-14), arms (Fig. 18-15), hands (Fig. 18-16), and other parts of the body. Wrinkling is reduced, pigmented lentigines are greatly reduced, and the skin texture is smoother. The skin appears more even in color and texture.

REFERENCES

1. Fitzpatrick TB. The validity and practicality of sun-reactive skin types I through VI. *Arch Dermatol* 1988;124:869–871.
2. Alster TS. *Manual of cutaneous laser techniques.* Philadelphia: Lippincott-Raven Publishers, 1997.

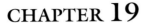

CHAPTER 19

PUTTING IT ALL TOGETHER

Achieving Optimal Results

▷ Achieving Optimal Results

We believe it is possible to obtain consistently good liposculpture results in all appropriate patients if all phases of the procedure are done in a consistent, methodical fashion. This takes the combined effort of all members of the surgical staff. The most important points to remember are:

▶ Choose the "right" patient with realistic expectations.
▶ Set realistic, achievable surgical goals.
▶ Thoroughly inform the patient of expectations, risks, and all aspects of the pre- and postoperative period.
▶ Be sure that the surgeon is adequately trained in the procedure being undertaken.
▶ Establish clear-cut procedures that are clearly understood and followed by nurses and other support personnel.
▶ Use tumescent solution with great care, paying particular attention to the amount of lidocaine infused.
▶ Perform surgical procedures consistently so as to produce reproducible results.
▶ Allow adequate time for each surgery, so that one is not rushed to complete the case because other patients are waiting.

Following a protocol such as this should give good cosmetic results, minimal postoperative problems, and certainly many fewer secondary procedures. The surgeon who adheres to these points will have satisfied patients and pride in his or her work.

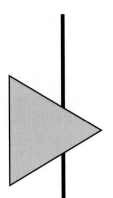

APPENDIX

Partial Directory of Liposculpture Apparatus Manufacturers

▷ Suction and Infiltration Pumps, Cannulas, Instruments, and Supplies

Bernsco Surgical Supply, Inc.
4055 23rd Avenue West
Seattle, WA 98199
Phone: (800) 231-8409
Fax: (206) 284-7859
www.bernsco.com

Byron Medical Inc.
602 W. Rillito St.
Tucson, AZ 85705
Phone: (800) 777-3434
Fax: (520) 746-1757
www.byronmedical.com

Wells Johnson
8000 South Kolb Road
Tucson, AZ 85731-8230
Phone: (800) 528-1597
Fax: (520) 885-1189
www.wellsgrp.com

▷ Smoke Evacuation Equipment

Buffalo Filter Co., Inc.
6000 North Bailey Avenue, Suite 9
Buffalo, NY 14226
Phone: (800) 343-2324
Fax: (716) 835-3414
www.buffalofilter.com

▷ Ultrasound Equipment

Bernsco Surgical Supply, Inc.
4055 23rd Avenue West
Seattle, WA 98199
Phone: (800) 231-8409
Fax: (206) 284-7859
www.bernsco.com

Rich-Mar
P.O. Box 879
Inola, OK 74036
Phone: (800) 762-4665
Fax: (918) 543-3334
www.richmar.web.com

▷ Lasers

Coherent Medical Group
3290 West Bayshore Road
Palo Alto, CA 94303
Phone: (800) 227-1914 or (800) 635-1313
Fax: (650) 857-0146
www.coherentmedical.com

▷ Miscellaneous Surgical Equipment

ValleyLab
5920 Longbow Drive
Boulder, CO 80301-3299
Phone: (800) 255-8522
Fax: (303) 530-6285
www.valleylab.com
Surgistat cautery units

Instrumentations Unlimited
93 South West End Boulevard, Suite 101B
P.O. Box 14
Quakertown, PA 18951
Phone: (800) 818-0094
Instruments

▷ Patient Supplies

Byron Medical
3280 East Hemisphere Loop
Tucson, AZ 85706
Phone: (800) 777-3434
Fax: (520) 746-1757
www.byronmedical.com
Surgical wear

Xomed
6743 Southpoint Drive North
Jacksonville, FL 32216-0980
Phone: (800) 874-5795
Fax: (800) 678-3995
www.xomed.com
Chin implant supplier

Hanson Medical Inc.
P.O. Box 1296
Kingston, WA 98346
Phone: (800) 771-2215
Chin implants

Implantech Associates Inc.
2064 Eastman Avenue, Suite 101
Ventura, CA 93003
Phone: (800) 733-0833
Fax: (805) 339-9414
Chin implant manufacturer

Body Support Systems
P.O. Box 337
Ashland, OR 97520
Phone: (800) 448-2400
Fax: (541) 488-5959
www.bodysupport.com
bodyCushion™

Design Veronique
P.O. Box 2263
Oakland, CA 94621
Phone: (800) 442-5800
Fax: (510) 569-2975
Chin straps

Mentor Corporation
P.O. Box 512228
Los Angeles, CA 90051
Phone: (800) 833-2237
www.mentorcorp.com
Surgical garments

Beiersdorf-Jobst, Inc.
5825 Carnegie Boulevard
Charlotte, NC 28209
Phone: (800) 537-1063
Fax: (800) 336-5578
www.jobst.com
Compression hosiery

▷ Medical Waste Disposal

Browning-Ferris Industries
P.O. Box 3151
Houston, TX 77253
Phone: (800) PICK-BFI
www.bfi.com

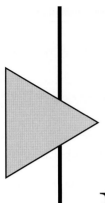

BIBLIOGRAPHY

▷ Tumescent Liposuction in General

American Society for Dermatologic Surgery. Guiding principles for liposuction, February 1997. *Dermatol Surg* 1997;23:1127–1129.

Apfelberg DB. Tumescent liposuction issues. *Dermatol Surg* 1997;23:401–402.

Asken S. The importance of accurate reporting on liposuction surgery to the public. *J Dermatol Surg Oncol* 1990;16:228–230.

Asken S. Perils and pearls of liposuction. *Dermatol Clin* 1990;8:415–419.

Clayton DN, Clayton JN, Lindley TS, Clayton JL. Large volume lipoplasty. *Clin Plast Surg* 1989;16:305–312.

Coleman WP 3rd. Liposuction and anesthesia. *J Dermatol Surg Oncol* 1987; 13:1295–1296.

Coleman WP 3rd. The dermatologist as a liposuction surgeon. *J Dermatol Surg Oncol* 1988;14:1057–1058.

Coleman W. Liposuction. In: Coleman W, Hanke C, Alt T, Asken S, eds. *Cosmetic surgery of the skin*. Philadelphia: BC Decker Inc., 1991:213–238.

Coleman WP 3rd. Fundamentals of good liposculpture technique. *J Dermatol Surg Oncol* 1992;18:215.

Coleman WP 3rd, Lawrence N. Liposuction. *Dermatol Surg* 1997;23:1125.

Coleman WP 3rd, Hanke CW, Cook WR Jr, Narins RS. *Body contouring: the new art of liposculpture*. Carmel, IN: Cooper Publishing Group LLC, 1997.

Colon GA. State of the art in liposuction. *Dermatol Surg* 1997;23:1190–1191.

Committee on Guidelines of Care. Guidelines of care for liposuction. *J Am Acad Dermatol* 1991;24:489.

Courtiss EH, Choucair RJ, Donelan MB. Large-volume suction lipectomy: an analysis of 108 patients. *Plast Reconstr Surg* 1992;39:1068–1082.

Dolsky RL. State of the art in liposuction. *Dermatol Surg* 1997;23:1192–1193.

Drake LA, Ceilley RI, Cornelison RL, et al. Guidelines of care for liposuction for American Academy of Dermatology. *J Am Acad Dermatol* 1991;24:489–494.

Fischer G. Liposculpture. 2. Evaluation of the patient for liposculpture. *J Dermatol Surg Oncol* 1991;17:741–743.

Fischer G. Liposculpture. 3. Surgical technique in liposculpture. *J Dermatol Surg Oncol* 1991;17:964–966.

Fischer G. Liposculpture. 4. Fundamentals of good liposculpture technique. *J Dermatol Surg Oncol* 1992;18:216–219.

Fischer G. Liposculpture. My technique. *Dermatol Surg* 1997;23:1183–1187.

Fournier PF. Who should do syringe liposculpturing? *J Dermatol Surg Oncol* 1988;14:1055–1056.

Fournier P. State of the art in liposuction. *Dermatol Surg* 1997;23:1189.

Gasprotti M. Superficial liposuction: a new application of the technique for aged and flaccid skin. *Aesthetic Plast Surg* 1992;16:141–153.

Goddio AS. Skin retraction following suction lipectomy by treatment site: a study of 500 procedures in 458 selected subjects. *Plast Reconstr Surg* 1991;87:66–75.

Grazer, FM, ed. *Atlas of suction assisted lipectomy in body sculpture*. New York: Churchill-Livingstone, 1992.

Hanke CW, Bullock S, Bernstein G. Current status of tumescent liposuction in the United States: National survey results. *Dermatol Surg* 1996;22:595–598.

Hetter GP. Closed suction lipoplasty in 1078 patients: Illouz told the truth. *Aesthetic Plast Surg* 1988;12:183–185.

Hunstad JP. Tumescent and syringe liposculpture: a logical partnership. *Aesthetic Plast Surg* 1995;19:321–333.

Illouz YG. Body contouring by lipolysis: A 5-year experience with over 3,000 cases. *Plast Reconstr Surg* 1983;72:591–597.

Illouz YG. Study of subcutaneous fat. *Aesthetic Plast Surg* 1990;14:165–177.

Lawrence N, Coleman WP 3rd. Liposuction. *Adv Dermatol* 1996;11:19–49.

Lewis CM. Lipoplasty in males. *Clin Plast Surg* 1989;16:355–360.

Lillis PJ. Liposuction surgery under local anesthesia: limited blood loss and minimal lidocaine absorption. *J Dermatol Surg Oncol* 1988;Oct 14(10):1145–1148.

Lillis PJ. The tumescent technique for liposuction surgery. *Dermatol Clin* 1990; 8:439–450.

Mladick RA. Ten commandments for safe lipoplasty. *Plast Reconstr Surg* 1991;87:382.

Moy R. Tumescent Liposuction Council bulletin: technical tips. *Dermatol Surg* 1997;23:214.

Narins RS. Liposuction and anesthesia. *Dermatol Clin* 1990;8:421.

Newman J. Training in liposuction for dermatologists. *Dermatol Clin* 1990;8:581–582.

Pitman GH. *Operative planning and surgical strategies: liposuction and aesthetic surgery*. St Louis: Quarterly Medical Publishing, 1993.

Pitman GH. Liposuction. *Dermatol Surg* 1995;21:441–447.

Skouge JW. The biochemistry and development of adipose tissue and the pathophysiology of obesity as it relates to liposuction surgery. *Dermatol Clin* 1990;8:385–393.

Stegman SJ. Technique variations in liposuction surgery. *Dermatol Clin* 1990;8:457–461.

Teimourian B, Fisher JB. Suction curettage to remove excess fat for body contouring. *Plast Reconstr Surg* 1981;68:50–58.

The American Society for Dermatologic Surgery. Guiding principles for liposuction. *Dermatol Surg* 1997;23:1127–1129.

Toledo LS. Syringe liposculpture: a two-year experience. *Aesthetic Plast Surg* 1991;15:316–321.

▷ History of Tumescent Liposuction

Coleman WP 3rd. The history of liposuction surgery. *Dermatol Clin* 1990;8:381–383.

Coleman WP 3rd. The history of liposculpture. *J Dermatol Surg Oncol* 1990;16:1086.

Field L. The dermatologist and liposuction: a history. *J Dermatol Surg Oncol* 1987;13:1040–1041.

Hanke CW, Coleman WP, Francis LA. History of dermatologic cosmetic surgery. *Am J Cosmet Surg* 1992;9:231–234.

Illouz YG. History and current concepts of lipoplasty. *Clin Plast Surg* 1996;23:721–730.

Klein JA. The tumescent technique for liposuction surgery. *Am J Cosmet Surg* 1987;4:263–267.

Klein JA. The tumescent technique: Anesthesia and modified liposuction technique. *Dermatol Clin* 1990;8:425–437.

Klein JA. Tumescent technique for local anesthesia improves safety in large-volume liposuction. *Plast Reconstr Surg* 1993;92:1085–1098.

Klein J. The two standards of care for tumescent liposuction [Editorial]. *Dermatol Surg* 1997;23:1194–1195.

▷ Tumescent Anesthesia

Alper MH. Toxicity of local anesthetics. *N Engl J Med* 1976;295:1432–1433.

Bennett PN, Aarons LJ, Bending MR, Steiner JA, Rowland M., et al. Pharmacokinetics of lidocaine and its deethylated metabolite. Dose and time dependency studies in man. *J Pharmacokinet Biopharm* 1982;10:265–281.

Coleman WP 3rd. Liposuction and anesthesia. *J Dermatol Surg Oncol* 1987;13:1295–1296.

Coleman WP 3rd. Tumescent anesthesia with a lidocaine dose of 55 mg/kg is safe for liposuction. *Dermatol Surg* 1996;22:919.

Coleman WP 3rd, Badame A, Phillips JH 3rd. A new technique for injection of tumescent anesthetic mixtures. *J Dermatol Surg Oncol* 1991;17:535–537.

Courtiss EH, Kanter MA, Kanter WR, Ransil BJ. The effect of epinephrine on blood loss during suction lipectomy. *Plast Reconstr Surg* 1991;88:801.

Covino BG. Systemic toxicity of local anesthetic agents [Editorial]. *Anesth Analg* 1978;47:387–388.

de Jong RH. Toxic effects of local anesthetics. *JAMA* 1978;239:1166–1168.

Hanke CW, Coleman WP 3rd, Lillis PJ, et al. Infusion rates and levels of premedication in tumescent liposuction. *Dermatol Surg* 1997;23:1131–1134.

Hetter GP. The effect of low-dose epinephrine on the hematocrit drop following lipolysis. *Aesthetic Plast Surg* 1984;8:19–21.

Kaplan B, Moy RL. Comparison of room temperature and warmed local anesthetic solution for tumescent liposuction. A randomized double blind study. *Dermatol Surg* 1996;22:707–709.

Klein JA. Anesthesia for liposuction in dermatologic surgery. *J Dermatol Surg Oncol* 1988;14:1124–1132.

Klein JA. The tumescent technique: anesthesia and modified liposuction technique. *Dermatol Clin* 1990;8:425.

Klein JA. Tumescent technique for regional anesthesia permits lidocaine doses of 35 mg/kg for liposuction. *J Dermatol Surg Oncol* 1990;16:248–263.

Klein JA. Tumescent technique for local anesthesia improves safety in large-volume liposuction. *Plast Reconstr Surg* 1993;92:1085–1098.

Klein JA. Tumescent technique chronicles. Local anesthesia, liposuction, and beyond. *Dermatol Surg* 1995;21:449–457.

Klein JA, Kassarjdian N. Lidocaine toxicity with tumescent liposuction. *Dermatol Surg* 1997;23:1169–1174.

Lillis PJ. The tumescent technique for liposuction surgery. *Dermatol Clin* 1990;8:439.

Lillis PJ. Liposuction surgery under local anesthesia: limited blood loss and minimal lidocaine absorption. *J Dermatol Surg Oncol* 1988;14:1145–1148.

Mather LE, Thomas J. Metabolism of lidocaine in man. *Life Sci* 1972;11:915–919.

Mladick RA. The effect of epinephrine on blood loss during suction lipectomy. *Plast Reconstr Surg* 1992;90:536–537.

McKay W, Morris R, Mushlin P. Sodium bicarbonate attenuates pain on skin infiltration with lidocaine, with or without epinephrine. *Anesth Analg* 1987;66:572–574.

Narins RS. Liposuction and anesthesia. *Dermatol Clin* 1990;8:421–424.

Narins RS, Coleman WP III. Minimizing pain for liposuction anesthesia. *Dermatol Surg* 1997;23:1137–1140.

Ostad A, Kageyama N, Moy R. Tumescent anesthesia with a lidocaine dose of 55 mg/kg is safe for liposuction. *Dermatol Surg* 1996;22:921–927.

Pitman GH. Tumescent technique in liposuction. *Plast Reconstr Surg* 1995;95:612–613.

Piveral K. Systemic lidocaine absorption during liposuction. *Plast Reconstr Surg* 1987;80:643.

Rohrich RJ, Beron SJ, Fodor PB. The role of subcutaneous infiltration in suction-assisted lipoplasty: a review. *Plast Reconstr Surg* 1997;99:514–519.

Samdal F, Amland PF, Bugge JF. Plasma lidocaine levels during suction-assisted lipectomy using large doses of dilute lidocaine with epinephrine. *Plast Reconstr Surg* 1994;93:1217–1223.

Stewart JH, Chinn SE, Cole GW, Klein JA. Neutralized lidocaine with epinephrine for local anesthesia, part II. *J Dermatol Surg Oncol* 1990;16:842.

Stewart JH, Cole GW, Klein JA. Neutralized lidocaine with epinephrine for local anesthesia. Part I. *J Dermatol Surg Oncol* 1989;15:1081–1083.

Stone A. Tumescent technique with local anesthesia for liposuction. *Plast Reconstr Surg* 1995;95:603–605.

▷ Ultrasonic Liposculpture

American Society for Dermatologic Surgery. Update from the Ultrasonic Liposuction Task Force. *Dermatol Surg* 1997;23:211–214.

Coleman WP III. Tumescent Liposuction Council bulletin: a primer on ultrasonic liposuction. *Dermatol Surg* 1997;23:211–212.

Cook WR Jr. Utilizing external ultrasonic energy to improve the results of tumescent liposculpture. *Dermatol Surg* 1997;23:1207–1211.

Cookrreria JA. Mixed liposculpture: aspiration and ultrasonic. *Am J Cosmet Surg* 1997;13:129–134.

Havoonjian HH, Luftman DB, Menaker GM, Moy RL. External ultrasonic tumescent liposuction: a preliminary study. *Dermatol Surg* 1997;23:1201–1206.

Igra H, Satur NM. Tumescent liposuction vs. internal ultrasonic-assisted tumescent liposuction. *Dermatol Surg* 1997;23:1213–1218.

Kloehn R. Liposuction with "sonic sculpture": Six years' experience with more than 600 patients. *Aesthet Surg Quart* 1996;16:123–128.

Kramer JF. Ultrasound: evaluation of its mechanical and thermal effects. *Arch Phys Med Rehabil* 1984:65:223–227.

Kuitert JF. Ultrasonic energy as an adjunct in the management of radiculitis and similar referred pain. *Am J Phys Med* 1954;33:61–65.

Lawrence N, Coleman WP III. The biologic basis of ultrasonic liposuction. *Dermatol Surg* 1997;23:1197–1200.

Maxwell GP, Gingrass MK. Ultrasound-assisted lipoplasty: a clinical study of 250 consecutive patients. *Plast Reconstr Surg* 1998;101:189–202.

Rohrich RJ, Beran SJ, Kenkel JM, Adams WP Jr, DiSpaltro F. Extending the role of liposuction in body contouring with ultrasound-assisted liposuction. *Plast Reconstr Surg* 1998;101:1090–1102.

Scheflan M, Tazi H. Ultrasonically assisted body contouring. *Aesthet Surg Quart* 1996;16:117–122.

Shiffman MA. Task force on ultrasound-assisted lipoplasty. *Plast Reconstr Surg* 1997; 100:1931.

Teimourian B. Ultrasound-assisted liposuction. *Plast Reconstr Surg* 1997;100:1623–1625.

Wells PNT. Surgical applications of ultrasound. In: Nyborg WL, ed. *Biological effects of ultrasound* (*Clinics in diagnostic ultrasound*, Vol. 16). New York: Churchill Livingstone, 1985:157–167.

Zocchi ML. Ultrasonic liposculpturing. *Aesthet Plast Surg* 1992;16:287–298.

Zocchi ML. Clinical aspects of ultrasonic liposculpture. *Perspect Plast Surg* 1993;7:153–174.

Zocchi ML. Ultrasonic assisted lipoplasty: technical refinements and clinical evaluations. *Clin Plast Surg* 1996;565–598.

Zocchi ML. Ultrasonic-assisted lipectomy. *Advan Plast Reconstr Surg* 1996;11:197–221.

Zocchi ML. Ultrasonic assisted lipoplasty. *Clin Plast Surg* 1996;23:575–598.

▷ Technical and Practical Considerations

Abramo AC. A device to protect the incision in performing liposuction. *Plast Reconstr Surg* 1994;94:743–744.

Carpaneda CA. Study of aspirated adipose tissue. *Aesthetic Plast Surg* 1996;20:399–402.

Chajchir A, Wexler EA. New model of liposuction cannula. *Aesthetic Plast Surg* 1985;9:101–106.

Chang KN. Surgical correction of postliposuction contour irregularities. *Plast Reconstr Surg* 1994;94:126–136.

D'Assumpcao EA. Cannula for liposuction. *Plast Reconstr Surg* 1984;74:731–732.

Gherardini G, Matarasso A, Serure AS, Toledo LS, DiBernardo BE. Standardization in photography for body contour surgery and suction-assisted lipectomy. *Plast Reconstr Surg* 1997;100:227–237.

Goodpasture JC, Bunkis J. Quantitative analysis of blood and fat in suction lipectomy aspirates. *Plast Reconstr Surg* 1986;78:765.

Greenberg G. Lipoplasty: the informed consent and medicolegal considerations. *Clin Plast Surg* 1989;16:375–379.

Hecht MC. Setting up a cosmetic surgery office (from a lawyer's point of view). *Am J Cosmetic Surg* 1988;5:113–116.

Hetter GP. Optimum vacuum pressures for lipolysis. *Aesthetic Plast Surg* 1983;8:23–26.

Kirwan L. Photographing patients for liposuction. *Plast Reconstr Surg* 1995;95:942.

Mandel MA. Blood and fluid replacement in major liposuction procedures. *Aesthetic Plast Surg* 1990;14:187–191.

Pitman GH, Holzer J. Safe suction: fluid replacement and blood loss parameters. *Perspect Plast Surg* 1991;5:79–89.

Raskin BI. Use of ABD pads in liposuction. *Dermatol Surg* 1997;23:404.

Trieger M. Practical guidelines to informed consent for the cosmetic surgeon. *Am J Cosmetic Surg* 1984;1:36–37.

▷ Complications and Safety

Alexander JM, Takeda D, Sander G, Goldberg G. Fatal necrotizing fasciitis following suction-assisted lipectomy. *Ann Plast Surg* 1988;20:562–565.

Barillo DJ, Cancio LC, Kim SH, Shirani KZ, Goodwin CW. Fatal and near-fatal complications of liposuction. *South Med J* 1998;91:487–492.

Benvenuti D. Postoperative headaches following large-volume suction lipectomies. *Plast Reconstr Surg* 1993;92:1423.

Bernstein G, Hanke W. Safety of liposuction: a review of 9478 cases performed by dermatologists. *J Dermatol Surg Oncol* 1988;14:1112–1114.

Bernstmas KD. Death following suction lipectomy and abdominoplasty [Letter]. *Plast Reconstr Surg* 1986;78:428.

Covino BG. Systemic toxicity of local anesthetic agents [Editorial]. *Anesth Analg* 1978;47:387–388.

de Jong RH. Toxic effects of local anesthetics. *JAMA* 1978;239:1166–1168.

Dillerud E. Suction lipoplasty: a report on complications, undesired results, and patient satisfaction based on 3511 procedures. *Plast Reconstr Surg* 1991;88:239–246.

Dolsky RL. Blood loss during liposuction. *Dermatol Clin* 1990;8:463.

Dolsky RL, Fetzek J, Anderson R. Evaluation of blood loss during liposuction surgery. *Am J Cosmetic Surg* 1987;4:257.

Drake LA, Ceilley RI, Cornelison RL, et al. Guidelines of care for liposuction for American Academy of Dermatology. *J Am Acad Dermatol* 1991;24:489–494.

Ersek RA. Severe and mortal complications. In: Hetter GP, ed. *Lipoplasty: the theory and practice of blunt suction lipectomy,* 2nd ed. Boston: Little, Brown, 1990:223–225.

Finkelstein F. Massive lidocaine poisoning [Letter]. *N Engl J Med* 1979;301:50.

Gargan TJ, Courtiss EH. The risks of suction lipectomy: their prevention and treatment. *Clin Plast Surg* 1984;11:457–463.

Hanke CW, Bernstein G, Bullock S. Safety of tumescent liposuction in 15,336 patients. *J Dermatol Surg Oncol* 1995;21:459–462.

Hanke CW, Lee MW, Bernstein G. The safety of dermatologic liposuction surgery. *Dermatol Clin* 1990;8:563–568.

Klein JA. Tumescent technique for local anesthesia improves safety in large-volume liposuction. *Plast Reconstr Surg* 1993;92:1085–1098.

Klein JA. The two standards of care for tumescent liposuction [Editorial]. *Dermatol Surg* 1997;23:1194–1195.

Klein JA, Kassarjdian N. Lidocaine toxicity with tumescent liposuction. *Dermatol Surg* 1997;23:1169–1174.

Mateu LP, Hernandez JJ. Cutaneous hyperpigmentation caused by liposuction. *Aesthetic Plast Surg* 1997;21:230–232.

Ovrebo KK, Grong K, Vindenes H. Small intestinal perforation and peritonitis after abdominal suction lipoplasty. *Ann Plast Surg* 1997;38:642–644.

Pitman GH, Teimourian B. Suction lipectomy: complications and results by survey. *Plast Reconstr Surg* 1985;76:65–69.

Pitman GH. Reducing blood loss associated with lipectomy. *Plast Reconstr Surg* 1993;91:962–963.

Rhee CA, Smith RJ, Jackson IT. Toxic shock syndrome associated with suction-assisted lipectomy. *Aesthetic Plast Surg* 1994;18:161–163.

Roberts HR, Adel S, Bernstein EF. Prevention of venous thrombosis and pulmonary embolism: consensus conference. *JAMA* 1986;256:744–749.

Samdal F, Amland PF, Bugge JF. Blood loss during liposuction using the tumescent technique. *Aesthetic Plast Surg* 1994;18:157–160.

Stone A, Rispler J. Scars at cannula sites for liposuction. *Plast Reconstr Surg* 1997;99:257–258.

Talmor M, Hoffman LA, Lieberman M. Intestinal perforation after suction lipoplasty: a case report and review of the literature. *Ann Plast Surg* 1997;38:169–172.

Teimourian B, Rogers WB. A national survey of complications associated with suction lipectomy: a comparative study. *Plast Reconstr Surg* 1989;84:628–631.

▷ Liposculpture of the Face, Neck, and Jowl

Aske S. The Face-lift-cervicofacial rhytidectomy. In: Coleman W, Hanke C, Alt T, Asken S, eds. *Cosmetic surgery of the skin*. Philadelphia: BC Decker Inc, 1991:335–354.

Aston SJ. Platysma muscle and rhytidoplasty. *Ann Plast Surg* 1979;3:529–539.

Aston SJ. Platysma-SMAS cervicofacial rhytidoplasty. *Clin Plast Surg* 1983;10:507–520.

Avelar J. Fat suction of the submental and submandibular regions. *Aesthetic Plast Surg* 1985;9:257–263.

Boskovic DM. Submental lipectomy with skin excision. *Plast Reconstr Surg* 1995;95:1129–1130.

Brennan HG, Koch RJ. Management of aging neck. *Facial Plast Surg* 1996;12:241–255.

Candiani P. Surgical approach to the infraorbital (malar) fat pad and composite rhytidectomy. *Plast Reconstr Surg* 1994;93:652–654.

Cardoso de Castro C. The anatomy of the platysma muscle. *Plast Reconstr Surg* 1980;66:680–683.

Cardoso de Castro C. Extensive mandibular and cervical lipectomy. *Aesthetic Plast Surg* 1981;5:239–248.

Chrisman B. Liposuction with facelift surgery. *Dermatol Clin* 1990;8:501–522.

Cook WR Jr. Laser neck and jowl liposculpture including platysma laser resurfacing, dermal laser resurfacing, and vaporization of subcutaneous fat. *Dermatol Surg* 1997;23:1143–1148.

Cooks J, Cinflone J. Facial lipectomy. *Aesthetic Plast Surg* 1981;5:107–113.

Duminy F, Hudson DA. The mini rhytidectomy. *Aesthetic Plast Surg* 1997;21:280–284.

Ellenbogen R, Karlin JV. Visual criteria for success in restoring the youthful neck. *Plast Reconstr Surg* 1980;66:826–837.

Farkas L, Hreczko T, Kolar J, Munro I. Vertical and horizontal proportions of the face in young adult North American Caucasians: revision of neoclassical canons. *Plast Reconstr Surg* 1985;75:328–338.

Farkas LG, Sohm P, Kolar JC, Katic MJ, Munro IR. Inclinations of the facial profile: art versus reality. *Plast Reconstr Surg* 1985;75:509–519.

Farkas LG, Kolar JC. Anthropometrics and art in the aesthetics of women's faces. *Clin Plast Surg* 1987;14:599–616.

Giampapa VC, Di Bernardo BE. Neck recontouring with suture suspension and liposuction: an alternative for the early rhytidectomy candidate. *Aesthetic Plast Surg* 1995;19:217–223.

Goode RL. Removing double chins—the role of submentoplasty. *West J Med* 1997;167:427–428.

Goodstein WA. Superficial liposculpture of the face and neck. *Plast Reconstr Surg* 1997;100:284.

Guerrerosantos J. The role of the platysma muscle in rhytidoplasty. *Clin Plast Surg* 1978;5:29–49.

Hamra S. Composite rhytidectomy. In: Rees T, LaTrenta G, eds. *Aesthetic plastic surgery*. Philadelphia: WB Saunders, 1994:708–721.

Kamer FM, Lefkoff LA. Submental surgery. A graduated approach to the aging neck. *Arch Otolaryngol Head Neck Surg* 1991;117:40–46.

Kamer FM, Minoli JJ. Postoperative platysmal band deformity. A pitfall of submental liposuction. *Arch Otolaryngol Head Neck Surg* 1993;119:193–196.

Knize DM. Limited incision submental lipectomy and platysmaplasty. *Plast Reconstr Surg* 1998;101:473–481.

Koch RJ. An overview of facial wrinkles. *West J Med* 1997;167:428.

Lambros V. Fat contouring in the face and neck. *Clin Plast Surg* 1992;19:401–414.

Lewis CM. Lipoplasty of the neck. *Plast Reconstr Surg* 1985;76:248–257.

Marino H, Galeano EJ, Gondolfo EA. Plastic correction of the double chin: importance of the position of the hyoid bone. *Plast Reconstr Surg* 1963;31:45–50.

Michalany Filho S. Neck rhytidectomy: aesthetic treatment variations. *Aesthetic Plast Surg* 1997;21:32–37.

Millard DR Jr, Pigott RW, Hedo A. Submandibular lipectomy. *Plast Reconstr Surg* 1968;41:513–522.

Mladick RA. Lipoplasty: an ideal adjunctive procedure for the face lift. *Clin Plast Surg* 1989;16:333–341.

Newman J, Dolsky RL, Mai ST. Submental liposuction with chin augmentation. *Arch Otolaryngol* 1984;110:454–457.

Park JI. Preoperative percutaneous facial nerve mapping. *Plast Reconstr Surg* 1998;101:269–277.

Perkins SW, Gibson FB. Use of submentoplasty to enhance cervical recontouring in face-lift surgery. *Arch Otolaryngol Head Neck Surg* 1993;119:179–183.

Renaut A, Orlin W, Ammar A, Pogrel MA. Distribution of submental fat in relationship to the platysma muscle. *Oral Surg Oral Med Oral Pathol* 1994;77:442–445.

Schoen SA, Taylor CO, Owsley TG. Tumescent technique in cervicofacial rhytidectomy. *J Oral Maxillofac Surg* 1994;52:344–347.

Shiffman MA. Superficial liposculpture of the face and neck. *Plast Reconstr Surg* 1997;100:552–553.

Teimourian B. Face and neck suction-assisted lipectomy associated with rhytidectomy. *Plast Reconstr Surg* 1983;72:627–633.

Topia A, Ferreira B, Eng R. Liposuction in cervical rejuvenation. *Aesthetic Plast Surg* 1987;11:95–100.

▷ Liposculpture of the Abdomen, Hips, and Buttocks

Apfelberg DB. The vast "waistland": a rediscovered area in liposuction. *Ann Plast Surg* 1994;33:237–240.

Avelar J. Fat suction versus abdominoplasty. *Aesthetic Plast Surg* 1985;9:265–276.

Baroudi R. Body contour surgery. *Clin Plast Surg* 1989;16:263–277.

Baroudi R, Ferreira CA. Contouring the hip and the abdomen. *Clin Plast Surg* 1996;23:551–572.

Baroudi R, Moraes M. Philosophy, technical principles, selection, and indications in body contouring surgery. *Aesthetic Plast Surg* 1991;15:1–18.

Bronz G. Lipoplasty of the abdomen and lateral thighs. *Ann Plast Surg* 1991;26:389–401.

Budo JA. Body sculpture: the words become reality. *Aesthetic Plast Surg* 1996; 20:489–493.

Carwell GR, Horton CE Sr. Circumferential torsoplasty. *Ann Plast Surg* 1997; 38:213–216.

Coffey RC. Plastic surgery of the abdominal wall. *Surg Gynecol Obstet* 1910;10:90–93.

Crestinu JM. Scarless infraumbilical abdominal lifting. *Plast Reconstr Surg* 1998;101:205–214.

Field LM. Liposuction reduction of the suprapubic area. *J Dermatol Surg Oncol* 1990;16:856–858.

Floras C, Davis PKB. Complications and long term results following abdominoplasty: a retrospective study. *Br J Plast Surg* 1991;44:190–194.

Grazer FM. Body contouring. Introduction. *Clin Plast Surg* 1996;23:511–528.

Grolleau JL, Lavigne B, Chavoin JP, Costagliola M. A predetermined design for easier aesthetic abdominoplasty. *Plast Reconstr Surg* 1998;101:215–221.

Guerrerosantos J. Secondary hip-buttock-thigh plasty. *Clin Plast Surg* 1984;11:491–503.

Hunstad JP. Addressing difficult areas in body contouring with emphasis on combined tumescent and syringe techniques. *Clin Plast Surg* 1996;23:57–80.

Illouz Y-G. Body contouring by lipolysis: a 5-year experience with over 3,000 cases. *Plast Reconstr Surg* 1983;72:591–597.

Mantse L. The importance of patient positioning in liposuction surgery. *Plast Reconstr Surg* 1996;98:1123–1124.

Matarasso A, Matarasso SL. When does your liposuction patient require an abdominoplasty? *Dermatol Surg* 1997;23:1151–1160.

Nguyen TT, Kim KA, Young RB. Tumescent mini abdominoplasty. *Ann Plast Surg* 1997;38:209–212.

Pinto EB, Indaburo PE, Muniz A da C, Martinez YP, Gerent KM, Iwamoto H, Miziara AC. Superficial liposuction. Body contouring. *Clin Plast Surg* 1996;23:529–548.

Ryan RF. Which patient needs the abdominoplasty? *Plast Reconstr Surg* 1982;82:437–443.

Schrudde J. Suction curettage for body contouring. *Clin Plast Surg* 1984;11:445–456.

Teimourian B, Fisher JB. Suction curettage to remove excess fat for body contouring. *Plast Reconstr Surg* 1981;68:50–58.

▷ Liposculpture of the Lower Extremities

Chamosa M. Suction lipectomy of the ankle area. *Plast Reconstr Surg* 1997; 100:1047–1052.

Chamosa M. Liposuction of the kneecap area. *Plast Reconstr Surg* 1997;99:1433–1436.

Ersek RA, Salisbury AV. Circumferential liposuction of knees, calves, and ankles. *Plast Reconstr Surg* 1996;98:880–883.

Fodor PB. Lipoplasty of the knees and anterior thighs. *Clin Plast Surg* 1989;16:361–364.

Franco T. Aesthetic surgery of the upper and lower limbs. *Aesthetic Plast Surg* 1980;4:245–256.

Grazer FM. Cellulite lysing. *Aesthetic Surg* 1991;11:11.

Guerrerosantos J. Secondary hip-buttock-thigh plasty. *Clin Plast Surg* 1984;11:491–503.

Lillis PJ. Liposuction of the arms, calves, and ankles. *Dermatol Surg* 1997;23:1161–1168.

Martin MC. Comprehensive liposuction of lower limbs: basic concepts. *Aesthetic Plast Surg* 1996;20:49–52.

Mladick RA. Lipoplasty of the calves and ankles. *Plast Reconstr Surg* 1990;86:84–93.

Mladick RA. Circumferential "intermediate" lipoplasty of the legs. *Aesthetic Plast Surg* 1994;18:165–174.

Nurnberger F, Muller SG. So-called cellulite: an invented disease. *J Dermatol Surg Oncol* 1978;4:221–229.

Pitanguy I. Aesthetic plastic surgery of the upper and lower limbs. *Aesthetic Plast Surg* 1980;4:363–372.

Reed LS. Lipoplasty of the calves and ankle. *Clin Plast Surg* 1989;16:365–368.

Regnault P, Daniel R. Secondary thigh, buttock deformities after classical techniques. *Clin Plast Surg* 1984;11:505–516.

Schweritz S, Braun-Fazco O. So-called cellulite. *J Dermatol Surg Oncol* 1978;4:230–234.

Shaer WD. Gluteal and thigh reduction: reclassification, critical review, and improved technique for primary correction. *Aesthetic Plast Surg* 1984;8:165–172.

Teimourian B, Adham MN. Anterior periosteal dermal suspension with suction curettage for lateral thigh lipectomy. *Aesthetic Plast Surg* 1982;6:207–209.

Vilain R, Dardour JC. Aesthetic surgery of the medial thigh. *Ann Plast Surg* 1986;3:176–183.

Wanatabe K. Circumferential liposuction of calves and ankles. *Aesthetic Plast Surg* 1990;14:259–269.

▷ Liposculpture of the Upper Extremities

Franco T. Aesthetic surgery of the upper and lower limbs. *Aesthetic Plast Surg* 1980;4:245–256.

Glanz S, Gonzalez-Ulloa M. Aesthetic surgery of the arm. *Aesthetic Plast Surg* 1981;5:1–17.

Lillis PJ. Liposuction of the arms, calves, and ankles. *Dermatol Surg* 1997;23:1161–1168.

Pitanguy I. Aesthetic plastic surgery of the upper and lower limbs. *Aesthetic Plast Surg* 1980;4:363–372.

▷ Liposculpture of the Chest

Abramo AC. Axillary approach for gynecomastia liposuction. *Aesthetic Plast Surg* 1994;18:265–268.

Balch CR. A transaxillary approach for gynecomastia. *Plast Reconstr Surg* 1978;16:13–16.

Becker H. The treatment of gynecomastia without sharp excision. *Ann Plast Surg* 1990;24:380–383.

Brenner P, Berger A, Schneider W, Axmann HD. Male reduction mammoplasty in serious gynecomastias. *Aesthetic Plast Surg* 1992;16:325–330.

Carlson HE. Gynecomastia. *N Engl J Med* 1980;303:795–799.

Eade GG. The radial incision for gynecomastia excisions. *Plast Reconstr Surg* 1974;54:495–497.

Huang TT, Hidalgo JE,Lewis SR. A circumareolar approach in surgical management of gynecomastia. *Plast Reconstr Surg* 1982;67:35–40.

Maillard GF, Scheflan M, Bussien R. Ultrasonically assisted lipectomy in aesthetic breast surgery. *Plast Reconstr Surg* 1997;100:238–241.

Mladick RA. Gynecomastia: Liposuction and excision. *Clin Plast Surg* 1991;18:815–822.

Nuttall FQ. Gynecomastia as a physical finding in normal men. *J Clin Endocrinol Metab* 1979;48:338–340.

Nydick M, Pustos J, Dale JH Jr, Rowson RW. Gynecomastia in adolescent boys. *JAMA* 1961;178:449–454.

Pitanguy I. Transareolar incision for gynecomastia. *Plast Reconstr Surg* 1966;38:414–419.

Rosenberg GJ. Gynecomastia: suction lipectomy as a contemporary solution. *Plast Reconstr Surg* 1987;80:379–385.

Samdal F, Kleppe G, Amland PF, Abyholm F. Surgical treatment of gynaecomastia. Five years' experience with liposuction. *Scand J Plast Reconstr Surg Hand Surg* 1994;28:123–130.

Simon BE, Hoffman S, Kahn S. Classification and surgical correction of gynecomastia. *Plast Reconstr Surg* 1973;51:48–52.

Williams CW. Adolescent breast maldevelopment: buying time with liposuction. *Aust N Z J Surg* 1993;63:983–984.

▷ Blepharoplasty

Adamson PA, Strecker HD. Transcutaneous lower blepharoplasty. *Facial Plast Surg* 1996;12:171–183.

Fedok FG, Perkins SW. Transconjunctival blepharoplasty. *Facial Plast Surg* 1996;12:185–195.

Kopelman JE, Keen MS. Lower eyelid blepharoplasty and other aesthetic considerations. *Facial Plast Surg* 1994;10:129–140.

Rosenberg GJ. Correction of saddlebag deformity of the lower eyelids by superficial suction lipectomy. *Plast Reconstr Surg* 1995;96:1061–1065.

▷ Laser and Chemical Peels

Alster TS. *Manual of cutaneous laser techniques.* Philadelphia: Lippincott-Raven Publishers, 1997.

Brody H. *Chemical peeling.* St. Louis: Mosby-Year Book, Inc., 1997.

Coleman WP 3rd, Futrell JM. The glycolic acid trichloroacetic acid peel. *J Dermatol Surg Oncol* 1994;20:76–80.

Fitzpatrick TB. The validity and practicality of sun-reactive skin types I through VI. *Arch Dermatol* 1988;124:869–871.

Fitzau, RG. Chemical peeling and aging skin. *J Geriatr Dermatol* 1994;2:30–35.

Moy LS, Murad H, Moy RL. Glycolic acid peels for the treatment of wrinkles and photoaging. *J Dermatol Surg Oncol* 1993;19:243–246.

Newman N, Newman A, Moy L, et al. Clinical improvement of photoaged skin with 50% glycolic acid. *Dermatol Surg* 1996;22:455–460.

Rubin MG. *Manual of chemical peels, superficial and medium depth.* Philadelphia: Lippincott-Raven Publishers, 1995.

Teikemeier G, Goldberg D. Skin resurfacing with the Erbium:YAG laser. *Dermatol Surg* 1997;23:685–687.

SUBJECT INDEX

Page numbers followed by *f* refer to figures, page numbers followed by *t* refer to tables.